Shirley Leonard's *With Each Passing Moment* is a treasure! I thoroughly enjoy her engaging style, fresh metaphors, and refreshing vulnerability. Shirley shares her journey of caregiving to offer insight and encouragement to readers who find themselves thrust into this bewildering world. Understanding the ambivalent emotions and all-consuming exhaustion that often cloud this experience, Shirley chooses her stories, Scriptures, prayers, and "Shirl's Sanity Savers" to give caregivers a quick boost from a compassionate companion who has successfully navigated this challenging passage of life.

— **Patti Souder**, Director of Montrose Christian Writers Conference, Montrose, Pennsylvania

To: Linda
From: Shirley
— in His grip —

WITH EACH
PASSING
**Help and Hope
for Caregivers**
MOMENT

Shirley E. Leonard

Shirley E. Leonard
"He is our Peace."
(Eph. 2:14)

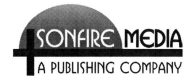
SONFIRE MEDIA
A PUBLISHING COMPANY

For information contact:

Sonfire Media, LLC
974 East Stuart Drive
Suite D, PMB 232
Galax, VA 24333

Cover & Interior book design by Larry W. Van Hoose

ISBN No. 978-0-9825773-8-7

Dedication

To my beloved Pilgrim, aka, The Rev.

You not only make it fun to be married, you also made it possible for this book to be lived out and written.

I truly do thank God for you.

Contents

Acknowledgments

Since this book has been supported in prayer by our extended family and our church families in so many places, over many years, there's no way to thank all who've helped. But I do want you to know how grateful I am to each one of you who've prayed or hugged or told me not to give up.

Special thanks also to the friends and faculty of Montrose Christian Writers Conference who've helped shape and hone my writing, especially Vie Herlocker, aka, The Book Mama.

Bless you all.

Introductory Note

Dear Reader,

I wrote *With Each Passing Moment* for you. Does your life ever whisper that you need comfort or hope? How about encouragement or wisdom? If you're a caregiver, life doesn't whisper, it shouts. You're expected to handle physical and emotional needs of somebody important to you, a role you probably didn't ask for and haven't been trained to handle. The rest of your life isn't stopping either.

Music was always important to my family—especially to my father. My dad loved to sing. He sang as he milked the cows, walked down the lane, or just when the mood struck him. He often sang silly songs, and sometimes, hymns. But his favorite song was "Twilight Time." [1] Although it was a love song, the message of being together at the end of the day became symbolic for me as I cared for my parents. In this book, I refer to the years of their needing care as the "twilight time ."

Music has always helped me cope. In the 1990s, when I was traveling to care for my parents, Wesley and Betty Ford, the car radio was set to show tunes, 60s rock and roll, or contemporary Christian stations— depending on my mood and which station came in where. But it was an old hymn that spoke to my needs as I struggled to be a good caregiver. The hymn, "Day by Day and with Each Passing Moment," was written in 1865 by a Swedish woman, Karolina ("Lina") Sandell-Berg. Lina had watched as her father fell overboard and drowned— while she could do nothing to save him. Perhaps out of her grief, she wrote a poem about trusting God during trials and tribulations. This poem became the lyrics to the hymn—the hymn that I went back to repeatedly during my parents' twilight time.

When my parents sank under waves of sickness, the process was slower than a drowning, but each change in them brought a grief of its own. To my surprise, blessings were tucked beneath the waves of this strange time, teaching me things I want to share.

The book you hold is part devotional, part memoir. It is arranged alphabetically by specific needs I experienced during the caregiving time. Stories from my life, scattered throughout the chapters, jump back and forth in time, reflecting the jumbled feelings and memories often triggered by a caregiving experience. Lines from Sandell-Berg's hymn provide hooks on which to fasten those memories, and are included in this book.

I've been a pastor's wife since the early 1970s. Dick's life and mine have been interwoven personally and professionally all that time, so many of these stories are his stories too.

In His Love,

Shirley (and the Rev.)

Day by Day and With Each Passing Moment

— Karolina Sandell-Berg

Day by day and with each passing moment
Strength I find to meet my trials here
Trusting in my Father's wise bestowment
I've no cause for worry or for fear
He whose heart is kind beyond all measure
Gives unto each day what He deems best
Lovingly, it's part of pain and pleasure
Mingling toil with peace and rest.

Every day the Lord Himself is with me
With a special mercy for each hour
All my cares He fain would bear and cheer me
He whose name is Counselor and Power
The protection of His child and treasure
Is a charge that on Himself He laid
As your days, your strength shall be in measure
This the pledge to me He made.

Help me then in every tribulation
So to trust Your promises, O Lord
That I lose not faith's sweet consolation
Offered me within Your holy Word.
Help me, Lord, when toil and trouble meeting
E'er to take, as from a Father's hand
One by one, the days, the moments fleeting
Till I reach the Promised Land.

With Each Passing Moment

CHAPTER 1

AND SO IT BEGINS

"Day by Day, and with Each Passing Moment"

But He said to them, "Why are you so fearful, O you of little faith?"
Then He arose and rebuked the wind and sea, and there was a great calm.
Matthew 8:26 NKJV

CONQUER ME AGAIN

Two days before Dad's stroke, I wrote in my journal, "Conquer me again, today, Lord Jesus, that I may be faithful to your calling."

Oh, brother. Did I really write that? It seems so grandiose now, or maybe just clueless. On that bright snowy day in January of 1990, I had no idea of the ways God would take me up on that naïve prayer over the next four and a half years.

Dad had his stroke on February 1. While in rehab after the stroke, he was diagnosed with lung cancer. At first Mom was Dad's primary caregiver. But when she developed both emphysema and clinical depression, she needed help. My sister, brother, and I—and our families—found ourselves in the middle of a world that was new for all of us: caregiving. It became a twilight time for the parents we loved so deeply. The long shadows of that world were frightening. We had to learn new skills to cope with unfamiliar situations. Some days nothing seemed sure except the fact that we had no idea what we were doing.

LAID-BACK CROONERS

Perry Como–now there was a dreamy singer! If you're rolling your eyes or shrugging your shoulders, it probably means you're too young to have any idea who he is, so let me fill you in.

Dad would be in his chair in the corner of the living room after supper and I'd be on the couch with my feet tucked under me, homework on my lap. It was time for the Kraft Music Hall and Perry was the host (1959 to 1967). The tiny TV screen would move off the commercial and this very relaxed guy in a sweater would come out and perch on a wooden stool. His opening song, "Dream Along with Me," always made us smile. Dad and I would make eye contact and we'd be ready to enjoy the hour of great entertainment.

The joke in those days was that Perry Como was so relaxed when he sang, you'd have to look closely to be sure he wasn't singing in his sleep.

That's how my Dad sang. Whether singing to the cows, singing on the tractor, or singing in the pickup as we delivered milk to Rayburn's Dairy, his voice was deep, sweet, and mellow.

Anyway, as I looked at Dad's face that week after his stroke, those memories rolled. I wanted Perry to come invite us to dream.

LEARNING CURVE

My knowledge of strokes was limited and inadequate. Early on, the damage seemed minimal. It wasn't. Those first days, I called from the New York hospital to my waiting, worried husband and daughters in Pennsylvania with rosy, unrealistic reports. Unfamiliar terms and procedures scared us all.

My sister, Carole, and brother, John, lived closer to home than I did but held full-time jobs. Their help was necessarily limited to mostly evenings and weekends. I was a pastor's wife and mother of three daughters, one still in high school. My life was full, but since I was technically unemployed, it seemed only right that I fill in as many days as possible.

As the oldest, I felt that I should at least have a clue about what needed to be done. Besides, I was a pastor's wife and these situations just came with the job. Dick and I were the ones everybody leaned on for comfort and strength in times of stress. What was the matter with me anyway? I felt like I should have had it all together and each time I didn't, the guilt and fear gremlins multiplied and their whispers in my head grew louder.

Soon the guilt and fear brought along annoying friends like impatience, resentment, and self-pity. As with all life challenges, good days and not so good ones tumbled over each other like yipping puppies. On the good days, I found myself suspecting that a bad one was just around the corner.

I began what was to become a biweekly, three-day schedule, traveling six hours round-trip. As stretched as I often felt, I became thankful for the unexpected bonus of time spent with my parents. I came to know Dad in a deeper way than ever before, and began a process of healing my relationship with Mom. (In many ways, she was the perfect mother. Without a doubt, we three kids knew we were loved. She read to us and often had cookies warm from the oven waiting when we got off the bus. But there were times when her drinking burst the perfect bubble and even now, long after her death, it's not easy to think about those times. Eventually, she overcame that crutch and her recovery was a blessing for all of us. But the drinking complicated our relationship, and although I loved her greatly, I battled hidden resentment and anger for many years.)

My siblings and I wanted to keep Mom and Dad at home as long as possible. This is the story of how we tried, with both victories and failures. The stress affected each of us in different ways. Our prayer is that in sharing our family's story, we can comfort others on this road, and show them they are not alone.

If you are in the middle of a situation like ours, my heart goes out to you. Some days will be awful. You may feel so drained and discouraged that you'll begin to wish somebody would put *you* in a "Home." Other days, you just might amaze yourself with a light spirit that lifts burdens all around you.

Keeping a journal helped me see things more clearly. It was a real sanity saver and much of this book comes from those pages. I also fell into the habit of leaving notes on my parents' pillows when I left New York to go back to Pennsylvania. My mom, an incorrigible pack rat, saved each one and some of them are included in this book as well.

So, dear caregiver, I know you're confused. I know you're tired. I know you're probably too busy to be reading this book! But if you can sneak a minute or two to do a little something to recharge your own batteries, my prayer is that *With Each Passing Moment* will be an encouragement for where you are, right now.

†·†·†

"Day by Day, and with Each Passing Moment"

God understands how fuzzy everything seems at this moment. He knows how frazzled you often feel. He also has the power to calm your jumbled thoughts, not just for this one moment, but also for each passing moment. Stop right now and let him.

Surely I have calmed and quieted my soul. Like a weaned child with his mother, like a weaned child is my soul within me.

Psalm 131:2 NKJV

Prayer: Open my eyes, Lord, that I may see what really matters today. Calm my fears and teach me to lean on you—day by day, and with each passing moment—until the answers come.

Shirl's Sanity Saver

Even if you've never wanted to before, start a journal today. Write down any part of this caregiving journey that has you stumped and simply wait for God to shed some light on that one thing. It may just create the calm oasis you need to keep going.

CHAPTER 2

When you Need...
AN ATTITUDE ADJUSTMENT
"Strength I Find to Meet My Trials Here"

For God maketh my heart soft.
Job 23:16 KJV

BAH HUMBUG

The countdown had begun. In just four hours, I had to get my act together, go be the pastor's wife, and smile. I didn't know if I could pull it off. It was Christmas Eve, 1992. I was about as jolly as a neat freak in a garbage dump.

My parents were critically ill and lived three hours north of our parsonage. Four hours to the west, Dick's mom was in the process of dying. Juggling trips to both places plus the needs of our kids and ministry had wiped us out. We were schizophrenic wishbones, pulled so hard in opposite directions that one more need would make us snap.

The people in our church family were wonderful. They were loving and kind and wanted to help. Unfortunately, they also expected us to be strong, steady, and full of faith, no matter what. At least, that's what I figured.

It was still too early to dress for the Christmas Eve church service so I clutched my ratty bathrobe with one hand and dialed the phone with the other. It was time to call in the reserves. There was only one person to call: Carolyn, my sister-in-Christ, and, like me, a pastor's wife. I dialed and waited for her to answer. Where was she?

Joy to the world, my eye. Scrooge was on the right track. All this merriment makes me mad. Why can't we just flip the calendar to April Fool's Day and admit that all is neither calm nor bright? Carolyn, please come home. If you're at the fabric store buying supplies to make lap robes, cut it out. If you're at the church, come home now. There is a mission field right here and the need is urgent.

The phone rang again. Then she answered. Finally, a glimmer of light in this bah humbug day.

I quickly dressed and went to her house. We talked. I cried, whined, and vented. She listened, cared, and prayed. I felt better than I had since Dick and I both had meetings canceled the same night. I went home thanking God for this holy interlude. In Carolyn's home, I could fall apart for a while, just long enough for my Creator to knit me back together again.

When it was time to go to the church service, I could hardly wait. And I couldn't stop smiling.

WAKE UP CALL

Chances are you picked up this book or someone gave it to you because in the middle of your already hectic life, you became a caregiver. Maybe today it just feels too hard. Perhaps a crisis slapped that label on you or maybe the role developed gradually, sneaking up on you before you realized what a big deal it was. Please believe me. You're not going crazy.

The whole thing was a surprise to me and I should have known better. After all, Dick and I had walked through plenty of caregiving mazes with people in our congregation. It floors me now to think I never suspected I'd be taking care of my parents one day.

As 1989 wound to a close, the whole world was changing. The Berlin Wall came down and Communist rule crumbled all over Europe. Dictatorships fell in South America and Noriega turned himself in to the Vatican. Political events in China and the USSR astonished even the most cynical observers. It seemed that God's Spirit was shaking events all over the globe.

Meanwhile, in our small corner of the world in a tiny town in Pennsylvania, God demonstrated his tender love to us in ways that were less flashy than revolution, but nonetheless real. Our three daughters: sixteen year-old Amber, nineteen year-old Carrie, and twenty-one year-old Mary, provided hectic but joyful challenges. Our two churches proved lively and exciting on many fronts.

Indeed, our cup was running over. On the surface, I felt fulfilled meeting needs in family and church. Yet underneath, a trickle of worry nagged at the corners of my mind. Something was wrong with my father.

Just before Christmas, Mom mentioned on the phone that Dad didn't seem to be quite himself. A couple of times he dropped a card while playing Euchre. Nothing major. After that, he felt like he was "getting the flu but it wasn't there yet." He didn't want to hear about going to the doctor.

"I'd feel silly," he'd reasoned. "What would I tell the doctor—that I think I'm *going* to get sick?"

Hindsight can be a cruel companion when it's coupled with regret. I wish we'd known more about TIAs[1], and if you don't know the warning signs, please stop now and read the information I've included in the notes section of this book. No one had any idea that something awful was about to happen to Dad, and to all of us.

But we were also about to discover God's ability to meet our needs in unforgettable ways. We were entering a completely new world.

THE HEDGEROW

I first learned the habit of praise on those long, quiet, childhood afternoons on our farm in the Finger Lakes region of New York. The hedgerow was my favorite spot and getting there was an adventure in itself. Even the walk down our lane filled me with anticipation as I trekked between rows of corn and then along the wheat field.

After I finally made it to the hedgerow between the last two fields, I'd take a while to get settled. First, I had to search out the exact spot under the trees and trample down the weeds to make a me-sized place. Then I stretched out on my back and gazed up at the leaf patterns above my head. Each time, changing shades of sky, trees, and clouds made it a new experience. My thoughts would drift: school, boys, family, friends, and always, I found myself talking to God. Mostly, I just whispered, "Thank you." My private retreat worked well for me through elementary school and into Jr. High.

MUD AND STARS

Then came a day of adolescent crisis. Mom was working late so I was doing supper dishes. Thinking over my terrible day at school, I indulged in crashing around pots and pans to vent my frustration. When I was done, I went out to sit on the front porch and sulk.

To my surprise, Dad was already there. We sat in silence. It had rained most of the day and I grabbed a stick leaning by the step and absently traced patterns in the soggy ground. Finally, Dad said, "What's wrong, honey?"

"Oh, Dad. This was the worst day of my life," I whined. I went on to describe the day's awful events. I failed an algebra test. My best friend was mad at me and I didn't know why. And worst of all, I saw my boyfriend walking another girl down the hall.

I ended this mournful litany with, "I feel as yucky and worthless as this stupid mud."

He didn't laugh. For a while, he didn't say anything.

Finally, he said, "Shirl, your problem is that you're looking in the wrong place. Look up and tell me what you see."

Until that moment, I hadn't even realized it was getting dark. When I lifted my eyes, I was amazed to see an incredibly lovely, star-filled sky. The clouds had all drifted away and galaxies sparkled above us. It was so beautiful that it brought tears to my eyes. In that moment, I was lifted out of my smallness into the vastness of God's handiwork.

"Life will always be full of both mud and stars," Dad said. "It's up to you where you set your sights."

✝·✝·✝

"Strength I Find to Meet My Trials There"

Remembering that moment, now that it was Dad's life in trauma, was just what I needed to shift my focus. I still had volumes to learn, but it was a start.

Fix your thoughts on what is true and good and right. Think about things that are pure and lovely and dwell on the fine, good things in others. Think about all you can praise God for and be glad about.

Philippians 4:8

Prayer: Father, the needs facing me feel huge today. Help me see them honestly but without being a drama queen (or king). Adjust my attitude, Lord.

Shirl's Sanity Saver

Pull up one happy memory. Write it down, or tell it to someone.

CHAPTER 3

When you Need...
COMFORT
"Trusting in My Father's Wise Bestowment"

What a wonderful God we have, he is the Father of our Lord Jesus Christ,
the source of every mercy, and the one who so wonderfully comforts and
strengthens us in our hardships and trials. And why does he do this? So
that when others are troubled, needing our sympathy and encouragement,
we can pass on to them this same help and comfort God has given us.
2 Corinthians 1:3-4

HUGS FROM NEAR AND FAR

The Thursday night of Dad's stroke, I drove to New York alone because Dick had an important church meeting. But he came on Sunday, bringing all three of our girls. I was so grateful for each of them; I needed them. We all needed them.

Mary said, "We weren't ready for this, Mom."

Carrie said, "I want to get him out of here. I just love him so much."

Amber said, "We miss you, Mom."

And Dick held me.

They were there all afternoon, filling me with strength and comfort.

I stayed; they had to go home. My cousin Ruthi called from New Jersey on Monday night. I couldn't believe it. I hadn't talked to her in so long and had no idea how she even knew about Dad. Her call was a huge blessing, like a warm hug for my spirit.

When we were kids, Ruthi was my buddy for "crazy-mixed-up-cousins'week." Her sister, Sharon, would come stay with my sister, Carole, and I'd go to Ruthi's house. There were seven kids in that house so there was always something fun going on.

When we grew up, Ruth and I even had babies the same night. Her Jeffrey and my Carrie were both born on January 16, 1970. All of that came back in a flash when I heard her voice and I suddenly felt grounded in the middle of what had felt like an out-of-control situation. She told me about nice things my mom had told hers about our ministry. It startled me to think maybe, just maybe, Mom was a little proud of me after all. It was a foreign idea but such a comfort at that moment.

THE POWER OF PRAISE

I'm grateful for my journals because without them, so much of what God was doing, as I faced the start of my parents' twilight time, would have sifted down through the cracks of my memory, lost forever. Journaling, for me, always starts with Scripture. One verse I read the day after Dad's stroke was an old favorite, but at that moment, it became a lifeline for my sinking spirit:

> **Whatever happens, dear friends, be glad in the Lord... Fix your thoughts on what is true and good and right. Think about things that are pure and lovely, and dwell on the fine, good things in others. Think about all you can praise God for and be glad about. (Philippians 3:1a; 4:8)**

Obeying that Word required a major shifting of gears in my head and heart. I had to force myself to quit fussing about the problems we were facing and focus on God's gifts to us.

Then I listed those gifts:

- I was home when Mom called about Dad's stroke. Considering our hectic lives, that was a gift.

- The ambulance came quickly and my cousin Eddie was on the crew. Having him there made Mom and Dad both much more comfortable.

- Mom and Dad's neighbor, Grace Ann, saw the ambulance and called Tarina, who lived just across the road. She came and prayed with them and took Mom to the hospital.

- My sister, Carole, and brother, John, were there for Mom and Dad very quickly, and then they were both downstairs to meet me with hugs and love when I arrived at the hospital several hours later.

- Dad could talk and even joke a bit. He kidded around about catching the stroke from Aunt Hilda, his sister. Then when a nurse asked to listen to his heart, he quipped, "What do you think it'll say?"

COMFORT MEASURES

Reading each of those entries warmed my heart but an even deeper comfort came during a more somber moment. After everyone else left, Dad let down his guard and admitted, "Getting a new hip was easier than this." His painful honesty tugged my heart but was somehow reassuring. He was still Dad.

The nurses had quite a time sorting out his mental state. When they asked him who the President was he said, "Moynahan." They were on the verge of writing "dementia" on his chart when he launched into a political commentary on why the country would have been better off with Patrick Moynahan as President. They chuckled, decided his mind was fine, and started working on the rest of him.

I stayed for a week but eventually I had to return to Pennsylvania and trust the hospital staff to take care of my father. That wasn't easy. Some of the nurses were tender and wonderful, but others were less so. A couple seemed downright mean. After just a few days, I convinced myself that nobody else could make Dad comfortable but me. Was that a coping mechanism or just plain arrogance? Whatever caused that grouchy attitude, I knew I had to get rid of it or I'd drive myself—and everyone at home—crazy. So as I drove to Pennsylvania, alone in the car with Jesus, we hashed it out. I vented. He listened.

That Sunday in church we sang "More Love to Thee, O Christ,"[1] and I was OK until a line in the third verse: "Let sorrow do its work, come grief and pain…"

I couldn't sing. The tears came without warning. Then Denny, our worship leader, sang "In His Presence." [2] His soothing tenor voice and the lyrics were so beautiful. I simply sat in the presence of Christ and let his peace and strength wrap around me. The Comforter had come.

†·†·†

"Trusting in My Father's Wise Bestowment"

The stresses of caregiving go deep. You may be trying to juggle a job, kids, and marriage, and you may feel like there's just not enough of you to go around. That's the time to accept his offer to carry the burdens too heavy for you. It's a good deal.

I, even I, am he who comforts you...

Isaiah 51:12

Prayer: *Lord Jesus, you truly are the Lord of all comfort. When I am all tied up in knots, come untangle me.*

Shirl's Sanity Saver

Do something nice for yourself. Take a long walk, or a hot bath. Have a good cry. Phone a friend and vent.

CHAPTER **4**

When you Need...
COURAGE
"I've No Cause for Worry or for Fear"

Yes, be bold and strong! Banish fear and doubt! For remember,
the Lord your God is with you wherever you go.
Joshua 1:9

TANGLED TRIALS

If only our troubles would learn some manners! They don't wait patiently in line so we can handle them one at a time calmly and efficiently. Fat chance. Too often, before we've caught our breath dealing with one urgent situation, new snags arise and demand our immediate attention. Complications pile up on each other in a chaotic bottleneck and none of the traffic signals work. We get scared.

The problems created by caregiving behave like bratty kids in the lunch line with no hall monitor around to take charge. They push at each other, vying for attention, making life miserable. It takes some pluck to look them in the eye and sort things out.

Have you ever been afraid of your own parents? I'm not talking to those of you who lived through the trauma of child abuse. I'm talking about another kind of fear altogether. It sneaks up on you little by little while the health of the people who raised you ebbs away to a place of no return. It leaves you drained of energy so often that the fatigue begins to feel normal, and that's when the fear begins. I was too scared to pull my car into their driveway. They were my parents. I loved them both. This was ridiculous. Somehow, I had to pull my act together. They were counting on me.

WHAT ARE YOU AFRAID OF?

Bravery has never been my strong suit. As a child, I remember being afraid of bumblebees, my mother leaving me, and sometimes, the dark. As a new bride, I found myself frightened by things that seem ridiculous now. I was nervous about lighting fires to burn trash, making business calls, and finding my way around in new places.

These fears gradually faded and were replaced by new ones as other responsibilities crept up on me. I had to learn how to be a pastor's wife and the thought scared me to pieces. Maybe it came from reading certain books. I thought a minister's wife had to wear pretty dresses and heels every day and keep a polished tea service ready. I was a jeans and sweatshirt kind of gal who had never used a tea service in her life, much less polished one.

Becoming a mother petrified me. My first pregnancy was filled with dreams of living in a huge house, hearing a baby crying somewhere, and not being able to find her. Growing older didn't help much. I was a wreck about becoming a mother-in-law and a grandmother. I had no idea how to do any of it right. All of those were just normal life stages, but still, each required a measure of confidence I lacked. Somehow, God always provided whatever courage I needed, just in time.

Then came the twilight time. But this was no Rod Sterling fantasy situation. This was real. Dad needed us, and Mom soon became overwhelmed with trying to cope with his needs. She wore herself out trying to protect each of us from becoming too burdened. We wore ourselves out trying to make it look easy.

PANIC PLACE

Much of the care became routine and there was no sense of needing any special bravery. Wheelchair transfers, radiation treatments, meds, laundry, adult diapers, wound care, oxygen, a nebulizer: all those things simply became facts of life. No big deal.

But then came the day I drove past their driveway. All the way the usual three hours north from Pennsylvania, I fought a nagging dread.

It's been many years since that day, but I can still remember the unbelievable terror I felt as I approached their driveway and realized I just wasn't ready yet to face them. The depth of their physical and emotional needs washed over me in a torrent. I drove on past the house and pulled off the road after about five miles. I was shaking and feeling so stupid. I sat there in the car, telling God how I felt, and asked him for the courage to face whatever was about to happen.

A GOOD TRADE

I clearly remember the gentle strength that began as a trickle and then steadily flowed into my heart and mind. By the time I turned the car around and headed back, I knew I could handle whatever waited for me. As it turned out, it was one of our best times together ever, even though some of it was very hard.

Thinking back, I see many other examples of God's gift of courage to me. Many of them I didn't recognize at the time, simply because I was so busy getting through one day after another. Juggling needs at home in Pennsylvania and at my parents' home in New York, I was often unaware of how frightened I was by all of it.

WES GETS BRAVE

Carrie and her husband named their first son Wesley, after my dad. Wes was and is a joy, but when he was little, his fear of loud noises drove me nuts. It didn't matter if it was a hair dryer or a chain saw. The good part was that it was a built-in safety measure because he wasn't tempted to run up to dangerous contraptions like many kids. But occasionally in the car, we'd have to take the long way around just to avoid some racket.

One crisp fall day, Carrie and the boys showed up while a new building project was going on at the old farmhouse Dick and I had been restoring for decades—and that we'll retire to after years of living in parsonages. Power tools were going and machines hummed but the almost ten-year-old Wes had no fear of any of it.

Courage came to Wesley gently, as a natural part of growing up. When he was twelve, he rode shotgun with me as we drove to the ER with his cousin, Raven, who was bleeding after hitting her head on the edge of an in-ground swimming pool. His steadiness gave me some needed courage that summer as he helped me with directions while we traveled unfamiliar streets.

God gave me courage when I needed it during the twilight time. Years later, he changed Wes from a fearful toddler to a young man of courage. You may need courage today just to admit that you're facing a very tough situation. It's hard to recognize that you're in over your head when you're trying to convince the world and yourself that everything is fine.

✝·✝·✝

"I've No Cause for Worry or for Fear"

Admitting you need help is a first step. Admitting you're scared is a good place to start.

> Be strong! Be courageous! Do not be afraid of them! For the Lord your God will be with you. He will neither fail you nor forsake you.
>
> Deuteronomy 31:6

> The Lord is my light and my salvation; whom shall I fear?
>
> Psalm 27:1

Prayer: *Father, I'm so scared. The situation in front of me seems way beyond my ability. And yet, even now I am beginning to sense your courage replacing the spaghetti in my backbone.*

Shirl's Sanity Saver

Write a list of the five things that scare you most today. Then lift them one by one in prayer.

CHAPTER 5

When you Need...
CREATIVITY
"He Whose Heart Is Kind Beyond All Measure"

Be glad; rejoice forever in my creation. Look! I will recreate Jerusalem as a place of happiness, and her people shall be a joy.
Isaiah 65:18

DAD, THE ARTIST

There's a picture in my mind of Dad in his wheelchair, hunched over an 11x14 inch "painting," sorting out markers, smiling. I love that memory. There weren't a lot of things that made him smile the first year after his stroke, but the art kits made him happy, at least while he was working on them.

One of our earliest needs was finding things to fill Dad's days. He was a guy who'd been both a dairy farmer and a factory worker. For quite a while, he was both. Even after he sold the farm and retired from the factory, he tended two huge gardens and a small fruit orchard behind their ranch house. He was always busy.

Being confined to a wheelchair was a huge jolt to Dad. Visitors provided a lift to his spirits, though; and family and friends came and brought food, love, and encouragement. But there were still too many hours to just sit.

I remember the day I stopped at a store on one of my trips to New York. I stood before a display of art supplies and wondered if Dad would like to try it. As kids, Carole, John, and I loved asking him to draw a picture of whatever. He always tried it and some of his sketches were quite good, at least, to his three junior art critics.

So when I found kits that didn't have any paint to spill, I was intrigued. There were markers and several different pre-printed pictures. By no stretch of the imagination could they be considered fine art but some of them were of farm scenes or forests, things very familiar to him. Why not try it? He loved it. A neighbor created frames for him. Making those pictures filled several hours a day for a while and helped us all cope. I still have several of the scenes he did and they bring me joy. The Father who created us evidently planted a need within us to create things too. Watching Dad work on those pieces made me appreciate that part of his plan.

BALANCING ACT

No one has ever accused me of being overly organized. Trying to balance things both at home and with my parents wasn't easy. Time, distance, and weariness were constant enemies to be tamed, and Dick and I needed some innovative ways to get through it all.

One of the biggest challenges was keeping our marriage on track. It was a tough time for us. We were already juggling two busy churches and three active, nearly grown-up daughters. The needs of our kids and our churches didn't stop just because we were going through our own traumas. Suddenly we found ourselves in the company of many sandwich-generation folks, coping with long-distance caregiving duties for our parents, as well as the complicated needs of our children. After years of it, the stress got to both of us. Our feelings were often so complicated that we had no idea how to talk about them. We tried. Sometimes, it helped and sometimes it didn't. We each had others we talked to, with the same iffy results.

OVERLOAD

Then the other shoe dropped. Dick's mom was diagnosed with terminal cancer. We were all shaken. Juggling the rest of our lives with the needs of my parents had already stretched us beyond anything we'd dealt with up until then. I wasn't sure how close our breaking point might be.

It was beyond scary. It was a nightmare, and yet, I can look back and see God's grace. Some days I was alarmed by my inability to handle both Dick's frustration and my own. Today I wonder why I ever expected that I could, or should. Now, from the distance of a few years, I feel like I'm finally getting a handle on what Dick and I were unintentionally doing to each other. I find myself wishing I could have understood then what seems so clear now. If we could have just learned how to listen to each other, it might have helped.

Listen to the people in your life. Really listen, with your total attention. It will make a difference.

JOURNALING JUNKIE

Finding time to pray was another challenge in those years. One way I created to cope was my journal. The process of writing out my jumbled thoughts and feelings became very therapeutic, plus, they became written prayers. I could pour out my thoughts to God on paper and feel both a release and his presence.

A few pages from my journal illustrate my seesaw feelings during that period:

Wednesday July 10, 1991

I will trust and not be afraid, for the Lord is my strength and song; he is my salvation. (Isaiah 12:2)

It's not easy to be married. Last night I wondered how many times that day Dick and I had each gone to you, Lord, for help in dealing with each other. The little things that drive us crazy are really dumb.

Thursday July 11, 1991

It may not be easy, but it's wonderful to be married.

Friday September 6, 1991

For the battle is not yours, but God's...Don't be afraid or discouraged. (2 Chronicles 20:15b,17c)

After the high places lately, yesterday was the pits. I read an article about a nurse who helped a family because she was so experienced in hard cases. Her insight changed them and it changed me. She told them that sick people are angry and they have to let it out somehow. Oh, Lord, how can that be such a revelation? But it is.

Dad's angry and it makes him demanding and narrowly focused and insensitive to Mom, to all of us at times.

Mom's angry, and it gets stuffed down over and over and she swallows oceans of tears to keep going and it becomes an undercurrent of depression and fatigue that sleep can't relieve.

And, oh, my own anger is what has made me so crazy lately. It surfaces over and over, and I get relief from you over and over too, but it's waiting to pop up some other way. I couldn't figure it out. Dick's great and the girls are great, but there's been this awful turmoil inside. I am finally beginning to realize that I'm angry too, so angry that my handsome, strong, happy-go-lucky father has changed into a helpless, needy stranger and that nothing I do can really change that. No matter how many sacrifices I make (or my family here has to make while I'm gone), I can never put things back. I'm angry with myself for not being able to get Dad to quit smoking sooner.

All these feelings are both irrational and normal, I suppose.

STUFFING THE TEARS

Back home with Dick and Amber, I wanted so much to be a happy, carefree wife and mom. They didn't need my sorrowful puss putting a damper on everything. Thoughts about what Mom and Dad were both going through plunked into my mind like a drippy faucet. It was annoying. I had to fight hard not to break down and cry, especially when the radio kept playing "Daddy songs."

Just when I almost lost it, the Scripture, "I can do all things through Christ who strengthens me" (Phil. 4:13), was just there in my heart, and it dried my tears and calmed me. Only God, who created all things, could create such tender, powerful ways for Dick and me to make it through those days.

As I write this, I look up to see a raccoon peering from a tree in one of Dad's paintings, reminding me of those precious days and of the Creator's loving care.

✝·✝·✝

"He Whose Heart Is Kind Beyond All Measure"

Don't you yet understand? Don't you know by now that the everlasting God, the Creator of the farthest parts of the earth, never grows faint or weary?

In the beginning, God created...

Genesis 1:1

Prayer: Ah, Creator, you have made us in separate and unique ways. Teach me again to laugh a lot, respect the other people in my life, and figure out new ways to cope. And if I need to scream sometimes, Father, please create just the right space and time for that too.

Shirl's Sanity Saver

Create something today: a meal, a letter, or anything you want. Give yourself credit for getting it done—whatever it is, and thank God for the strength to do it.

CHAPTER 6

When you Need...
DIRECTION
"Gives unto Each Day What He Deems Best"

Tell me clearly what to do, which way to turn.
Psalm 5:8c

LOST AND FOUND

My reputation for being directionally challenged began my freshman year at Lycoming College in Williamsport, Pennsylvania, when I walked downtown to shop at Woolworth's. Everything I needed was there and all of it on sale so I was feeling quite proud of myself, until I walked a block away from the store and suddenly nothing looked familiar. I walked a few blocks in each direction, growing more and more confused. Finally, I found a pay phone and called Karen, my roommate. I confessed I was hopelessly lost and heard giggling in the background. My roommates and suitemates were all from much larger places than Holcomb, New York. They thought it was hysterically funny that I could get lost just a few blocks from the college. The four of them trooped down to fetch me and even though I was thoroughly embarrassed, I felt their affection and we paraded back to Rich Hall in high spirits.

God has come to fetch me more than once when I've become lost in a maze of emotional or spiritual confusion. In the early years, I needed his direction to find my way to Jesus. Later, I needed his help to get my bearings when it felt like there were too many people needing too many things from me. I needed his guidance to show me what needs he was truly calling me to take care of and what I should let go of.

WAY TO GO, KING J.!

Something that helped me depend on God when I was "lost" was a story tucked in 2 Chronicles in the Old Testament about King Jehoshaphat. Maybe his story will help you too. King Jehoshaphat was not someone we normally learn about in Sunday school with Noah or Moses, but maybe he should be. He's actually listed in the genealogy of Jesus along with his father, grandfather, and grandson (Matthew 1: 7-8).

The Old Testament tells a fascinating story of his family tree. Today, the talk shows might say that King Jehoshaphat came from a long line of an old dysfunctional family. You can trace the pattern back through his father and grandparents and find a seesaw of good and evil balancing precariously on their family tree. This ruler had a few strikes against him from the get-go. Maybe you feel like you do too.

But he was no fool. He realized early in his reign as King of Judah that he needed to be true to himself, and for him that meant being bold in following God.

After living and reigning for many years, King Jehoshaphat came to a place that threw him for a loop. Not one, but three huge armies declared war on him at the same time.

I don't know what enemies you might be facing right now, but I'll bet you have more than just one. They might include illness, loneliness, weariness, anger, or something so deep that you haven't even formed it into words, but you know there's something wrong that you need to deal with. When we need direction, there is still no better place to go than the Word of God.

When Jehoshaphat learned about the triple threat of those armies ganging up on him, he did the best thing he could have done. He made a conscious choice to turn his heart to the Lord. It would have been understandable if he walked away in a huff of resentment. Or he might have bluffed his way through in a macho attitude that said, "I've handled bullies before and I can handle these thugs by myself." But he didn't. Instead, he admitted he was really quite helpless in the face of the combined military might of three great powers. He prayed, "We don't know what to do, but we are looking to you, Lord" (2 Chronicles 20:12).

NOT YOUR BATTLE

God didn't leave Jehoshaphat hanging. He sent His Holy Spirit to speak through one of the men there. It was the prophet Jahaziel who delivered the memorable words, "The battle is not yours, but God's" (2 Chronicles 20: 15). He went on to tell Jehoshaphat that, "You won't need to fight. Take your places; stand quietly and see the incredible rescue operation God will perform for you. Don't be afraid or discouraged" (vs. 16-17).

Then the King fell before the Lord in worship and all the people of Jerusalem followed suit. The next morning they went out, not to surrender to the enemy or do battle, but to praise and worship the

Creator, the God of the universe. The Bible says that the moment they began to sing and praise, the Lord caused those three armies to fight and destroy each other (2 Chronicles 20: 22 -23).

✝·✝·✝

"Gives unto Each Day What He Deems Best"

You can pretend this business of caregiving is no big deal. You can let yourself believe that everything depends on you. You can put on a sunny face and hide the confusion inside. Or, you can admit to God that you really don't have a clue what to do about your situation, but you trust that he does know.

In everything you do, put God first, and he will direct you and crown your efforts with success.

Proverbs 3:6

Prayer: Lord, where I'm lost, point me in the right direction. Where I've wandered off, set me back on the right path.

Shirl's Sanity Saver

Try thinking about the Bible as your personal GPS, and turn to it, expecting the Holy Spirit to direct your way.

CHAPTER 7

When you Need...
ENCOURAGEMENT
"Lovingly, It's Part of Pain and Pleasure"

I will answer them before they even call to me. While they are still talking to me about their needs, I will go ahead and answer their prayers.
Isaiah 65:24

LIFE LESSONS

I had a reputation in high school. (No, not that kind of reputation!) I was known for two things: for being the shortest girl in the class and for being a lousy speller. I couldn't do much about being short, but I did decide to work on my spelling. (That was a long time before spell-checkers.)

Then we had an assignment in English to write about an object, anthropomorphically. Big words always intrigued me and this one sounded like fun. Give a thing a personality. OK. I could do that.

I have no memory at all of what I wrote about in my essay, but more than forty years later, I still remember a classmate's composition. He stood straight and confident as he read, "I Am a Pencil." He amazed me with what seemed at the time to be incredible insights into what it must be like to be made of graphite, and used and abused by a variety of people. I was impressed. More than that, I was moved. Then the teacher shot him down with a scathing critique of his technical mistakes. (We had to hand in copies before class.) I remember my friend's face. I knew he was hurt, disappointed, and probably angry, but he did a remarkable job of keeping his composure. Any pencil would have been proud.

I remember thinking that if I were a teacher, I'd make sure to grade on two levels: technical merit and content. I'd never allow a student to think his writing was worthless because of spelling or grammar or sentence structure. I'd be sure to look deeper. I loved thinking about how encouraging my words could be.

I didn't become a teacher. But lately I've realized that our incredible Lord Jesus, our Master Teacher, has looked way beyond my technical mistakes. His mercy has covered me like a blanket, and he has looked deeply into my heart. I've messed up so often and so badly. I've earned a D minus at best many days in terms of attitude and action. He looks at me with compassion instead of condemnation and that makes all the difference.

Any good English teacher must stress the importance of correct grammar and proper sentence structure. It's important to spell correctly. I'm grateful for the teachers I had who taught me to diagram a sentence. But I'm even more grateful for the encouragement I received to express my thoughts and to find joy in that expression.

Belonging to Christ carries responsibility for obedience and faithfulness. But when I blow it, I'm so very grateful for his grace, reminding me that when I mess up, he doesn't reject me.

It's not that he tolerates sloppiness. It's that, I am still not all I should be… but, forgetting the past, and looking forward to what lies ahead, I press on…

(Philippians 3:13 and 14a)

For My yoke is easy and My burden is light.

(Matthew 11:30 NKJV)

I'm still not a great speller. I'm still short. But I'm loved by the author of life. Life is good.

MICHAEL AND THE YOKE

Encouragement can come to us in lots of ways, and from some delightfully surprising people, and age seems to be no barrier.

"What's a yoke for, Grandma?" asked Michael. He was two. We were cuddled on the couch reading a story and there was a picture of an ox. He didn't ask about the strange-looking animal, only the yoke. You couldn't even see any yoke. I only mentioned that sometimes oxen wear them and he wondered what they were for. At two.

Jesus drew us a word picture of a yoke that we can't see with our eyes either. I know in my head what it's for. It's supposed to keep my life in balance. But sometimes, actually, a lot of times, I forget about it. I push through my life, my work, my relationships, under my own steam, wearing myself ragged with self-imposed expectations that he never intended me to carry.

PERFECT FIT

I'm so glad Jesus doesn't say, "Hey, Shirley, come on and twist your neck into this contraption that will force you to perform perfectly."

He never chides me saying, "You goof-ball. You messed up again." He never once has shouted at me, "Hurry up and be better."

Instead, he sends the Holy Spirit to encourage me. He provides that sweet, persistent inner nudge, to accept the yoke. He bids me stop and relax into his embrace and quit making such a big production out of life.

†·†·†

"Lovingly, It's Part of Pain and Pleasure"

If your own life has been wearing you out lately, I invite you to slip into the yoke carved especially for you by the Master Carpenter. It just might make all the difference.

Come to Me, all who are weary and heavy-laden, and I will give you rest. Take My yoke upon you and learn from Me, for I am gentle and humble in heart, and you will find rest for your souls. For My yoke is easy and My burden is light.

Matthew 11:28-30 NASB

When I pray, you answer me, and encourage me by giving me the strength I need.

Psalm 138:3

Prayer: Lord, I have been so discouraged lately. You know. You see the weariness that fills my body and my spirit. Thank you for every small bit of encouragement you provide for the journey.

Shirl's Sanity Saver

Take a deep breath and just whisper, "OK, Lord. I'm ready to let you bear the burdens that are just too heavy for me."

CHAPTER **8**

When you Need...
ENDURANCE
"Mingling Toil with Peace and Rest"

He will give you the strength to endure.
2 Corinthians 1:7b

PETERING OUT

We were only about half way through Mom and Dad's twilight years when I hit the wall. I thought of an old, widely circulated, anonymous poem that said, "My get up and go got up and went." That's exactly how I felt.

On the Tuesday before Ash Wednesday in 1992, I read, "So take a new grip with tired hands, stand firm on your shaky legs, and mark out a straight, smooth path for your feet, so that those who follow you, though weak and lame will not fall and hurt themselves, but become strong" (Hebrews 12:12).

Those charged with caring for loved ones often come to a place where it seems impossible to go on. Enough, all ready, we think. And when one caregiving situation becomes tangled up in another, it can be a real mess.

DOUBLE TROUBLE

Caring for Mom and Dad had to take a back seat at one point. My wonderful husband was dealing with unrelenting shoulder pain and had an appointment scheduled with the doctor. I was with Mom and Dad, but planned to drive home for Dick's appointment. The day before I was to leave, Mom decided Dad needed an outing to cheer him up. I bundled him into his coat, got him settled in the wheelchair, and off we went to run errands. The ramp that was dry when we left was covered with ice when we got home. On her way out to help us, Mom slipped, fell hard—and broke her wrist.

Neighbors Sam and Rosie were alerted by their little dog, Maggie, who started barking frantically. Rosie stayed with Dad so I could take Mom to the hospital. In the emergency room, Mom said, "Life's not fair, but God is good." It was a truth to hold onto. But all I could think of as we waited for the doctor to set her wrist was, I love her, but no matter what, I am going to be with Dick for his appointment tomorrow. And I was.

Dick's diagnosis was "sympathetic reflexive neuropathy." It seemed like a mouthful when the doctor said it and it was as hard to deal with as to pronounce. We had thought his shoulder was dislocated. Instead, the doctor told us it was a complication from a recent hand injury. We faced weeks of appointments with neurologists, hand specialists, and finally, a long process of outpatient physical therapy followed by therapy to do at home.

One time during home therapy, Dick insisted I "push, push, higher, higher," lifting his arm. I made the mistake of looking at his face. The pain I saw etched there started my own tears flowing, for him. So we held each other a while. Later, I wrote in my journal, "In all our pain, you long to hold us close, too, Lord Jesus."

Lina Sandell-Berg was on to something when she penned the part of the hymn that says God's loving plan for us is found in "mingling toil with peace and rest." Our farm, the home that Dick and I had purchased years before, always provided a "rest for our souls," a time away from the parsonage and the daily responsibilities we had there. We needed a week at the farm as we adjusted to Dick's diagnosis and home therapy routine, so that's where we headed. It was more than a time of physical rest for Dick's arm; it was a week of reconnecting as husband and wife. We talked about how high our stress levels were. And yet, despite the pain and uncertainty, God amazingly renewed our romance and cemented our commitment to each other.

CARRIE'S CALL

One of my most vivid examples of endurance has been Carrie Dawn. She's our middle daughter, the birth order position that is said to be invisible, neither babied like the last born, nor leaned on like the eldest. Those generalities could hide a smidgen of truth, but they don't tell the whole story. At least not for our family.

Carrie had been so shy as a little girl that she didn't talk to her kindergarten teacher until January. She outgrew that stage and collected a group of friends wherever we lived as we moved from parsonage to parsonage. She was usually bubbly and full of fun. She graduated from high school and went away to secretarial college. She was enjoying life at college and living in an apartment with another student. But her life changed forever one quiet Maundy Thursday.

Dick and I were preparing for the evening church service when I answered the phone and heard Carrie crying. Then she said, "Mom, I have it." I guessed that what she had was Type 1 Diabetes. She was nineteen and had been losing weight for weeks. She hadn't seemed herself and I'd worried aloud about the possibility of diabetes, even though we had no family history. She assured me that a health-screening test had been negative. But tests can be wrong.

We marveled at her courage when she had to immediately adjust to giving herself four shots a day. She did that for years and then graduated to an insulin pump, which is part of her routine now. But she never let her diabetes be an obstacle or an excuse for embracing God's plan for her life. She fell in love with and married Jim, a wonderful guy. They have two delightful sons, Wesley and Michael. Her family moves from one sports season to the next and she loves it all, and runs marathons herself.

She and I went to a retreat together a few years ago, and while I sipped my coffee in our room, she was out for a run—in the rain—at 6:30 a.m.! Each time I watch her deal with the on-going challenges of her condition, I thank God for the grace she has to endure. Her faith is deep and she teaches me lessons of the spirit I need very much.

Carrie and her sisters helped me endure the twilight time with Mom and Dad, so many times, in so many ways. Just when I started to wonder how I'd make it through one more crisis, one more hassle, one of our daughters would call or write, and God would do it again. He'd give me what I needed.

BLESSED QUIETNESS

And then there were the private moments of deep connection with Christ that helped me endure. So often, in the car, coming and going between New York and Pennsylvania, where I'd been on automatic pilot through the details of caregiving or pastor's wife stuff, heading back to one or the other life, it would happen. I'd be luxuriating in the car with no other person, free at last to vent, relax, and collapse in the everlasting arms of Christ. I found myself drinking lustily from the living water, taking huge gulps to soothe the parched places in my spirit. Sometimes the radio was on and praise music washed over me like a healing blanket. Other times, the silence itself was a love song from heaven.

†·†·†

"Mingling Toil with Peace and Rest"

The power to endure doesn't come because we're especially tough or resilient or because we have a high tolerance for stress. It comes as a gift, simply because our Father knows we need it.

Let us run with endurance the race that is set before us.

Hebrews 12:1 NASB

Prayer: Father, it feels like I have nothing left to give. Renew me. Refill me. Restore me; help me endure. I'm Yours, Lord. Keep me going for however long this takes.

Shirl's Sanity Saver

Grab your journal and scribble down all the things that have drained you today.

CHAPTER **9**

When you Need...

FAITH

"Every day the Lord Himself Is with Me"

... all we need is faith working through love
Galatians 5:6b

TURNING POINT

The crisis snuck up on me. In 1971, I had everything in life to be happy about—a great husband, two adorable daughters and loving parents, but I was empty, miserable, and terrified. No one knew that in the long hours when I was home alone with our two little girls, I was quickly sliding into the unthinkable trap of hurting them. I never actually did, but I came close enough to scare myself. The war inside was seen only by God. Something had to change, and I thought I knew what I needed to do. In my mind, I had three choices. I could get pregnant again and have a boy. I could go back to college and finish my degree. I could get a good job with my nameplate on the desk.

I didn't need all of them. Any one of them would make me feel better about myself, and then I'd be nicer to the girls. It seems so ridiculous now, but that's what I really thought. I look at each of those points today and wonder how in the world I ever could have believed such nonsense. Here are my amateur stabs at self-analysis:

Each time I got pregnant, Dick had teased me that if I didn't have a son, he'd leave us both at the hospital. I knew that he didn't mean it, but some corner of my mind must have bought into the whole thing. I felt that Mom was very disappointed when I didn't finish college. I don't remember ever thinking Dad felt that way, and she probably didn't either, but in my head, I had let her down.

And the job thing was far-fetched. I suppose I'd seen movies where some well-dressed, smart-looking actress played the part of a woman executive who sat behind a brass nameplate at a big desk. To my silly young brain, that probably seemed like success.

My career goals had ranged from being a writer to becoming a professional dancer. By the time I was twenty-three, my job credits included working in a factory, clerical work in college, and working in a shoe store. I wasn't very good at any of them. No writing prospects, no dancing either. What a dud I was.

And I figured I wasn't cut out to be a mother either, because I was making a mess of that too. I must need something. I had no idea that what I needed wasn't a something but a *someone*.

That day in 1971, through a series of events that only God could have orchestrated, I found myself at a concert in a Lutheran church in Canandaigua, New York. This Methodist girl sat in a back pew, glowering at the college kids from Kansas who sang so beautifully. My younger brother, John, had talked me into going. He had no idea how that night would change the life of his big sister.

Compared to the college kids on stage, I felt ancient and very unattractive. They had perfect faces and figures and even perfect teeth. I hated their guts. They made me crazy with their songs all proclaiming, "Jesus is the answer." I was pretty sure they didn't even know the questions. They'd never had two little ones crying at the same time, needing more than anyone could give, or at least more than I knew how to give.

After the concert, I had a lengthy conversation with three of those annoying college girls. I told them the condensed version of my pitiful life and my list of three things that might fix it. One of the girls said, "Shirley, you've taught Sunday school and majored in religion in college. You know a lot about Jesus, but do you know him?" No one had ever told me there was a difference. Suddenly, it all made perfect sense. He was a real, live person, not a theory or vague idea. The way they prayed got my attention. No fancy words. They just talked to Christ as if he were right there in the room with us. So I did too. It felt very natural and the simplicity of it all was refreshing after all the years I'd complicated everything. That night I gave myself to Jesus and he began to change my life in deep and wonderful ways. That was the night faith was born in my heart.

But years later, when Jesus asked me to have faith about Dad's situation, it seemed too hard.

DAD'S AWAKENING

It must have been sometime in 1965 when I first started arguing theology with my father. That was ironic, because he never went to church unless one of us was in a special program or someone he knew was getting married or buried. Dad used to joke that he knew something God couldn't do. Then he'd grin and say, "God can't make a rock so big that he can't move it." When I tried to explain that his sentence violated laws of logic, he'd shrug it off and launch into a story about how he almost tipped the tractor over trying to pull out a huge stone in the back field.

Taking care of my father sometimes felt like a rock too big for God himself to move. It wasn't the work or even all the time away from my family so much as the sorrow of watching Dad's face contort in frustration over something he couldn't do anymore.

And yet—there were glimmers of God's work in Dad's heart that warmed mine. When he first came home from the hospital, we set up a bed in the living room and I slept on the couch to be close in case he needed help in the night.

I remember the chill that gripped my heart the night he called me to him and asked me to hide his gun. He kept it propped up in the corner of the dining room so it would be handy for chasing off rabbits or groundhogs from his garden. He looked at me with those beautiful blue eyes and said, "Shirl, I don't know how I'd ever get out of this bed to reach the gun, but I'm afraid of what I'd do if …." and then we were both crying. I remember how heavy the thing felt as I carried it to the cellar. I remember praying, or maybe it was more of a yelp in my spirit. By the time I got back upstairs, he was asleep and we never mentioned it again.

At rehab, a nurse's aide witnessed to Dad. A few days after that, my sister, Carole, called me. She said, "Guess what Dad asked me today! He said, 'What's this stuff about being born again? Is that something important?'"

So, over the course of many weeks, Carole and I talked to him. Neighbors Grace Ann and Burgie also talked to him. And then came the beautiful spring day when Dad and I were in the backyard. I was sitting on the grass in front of his wheelchair, leaning on his legs when suddenly he sat up straighter and said, "I think I get it now." We talked a long time, about who Christ is and what he'd done for us and of how much we needed him. Then, we prayed and cried and Jesus was there.

✝·✝·✝

"Everyday the Lord Himself Is with Me"

From the day he "got it," whenever Dad added a note to the letters Mom wrote to me, he'd write on the bottom of the page, "Count your blessings, Shirl," So I did. You can too.

And Jesus said to the woman, "Your faith has saved you; go in peace."

Luke 7:50

Prayer: Lord Jesus, there is much I don't understand. I do realize, though, that I am powerless to handle life apart from you. Increase my faith, Lord.

Shirl's Sanity Saver

Make a list. Count your blessings. Read them one by one and feel your faith grow.

CHAPTER 10

When you Need...

FORGIVENESS

"With a Special Mercy for Each Hour"

Be kind to each other, tenderhearted, forgiving each other,
just as God has forgiven you because you belong to Christ.
Ephesians 4:32

THE MUSTARD SEED NECKLACE

It felt like the elastic of my life had snapped, and in my limpness, the last thing I wanted was conversation.

> *Yikes, Lord! They expect me to be warm and winsome and I can hardly manage wimpy and washed out. Why did you bring me here anyway?*

> *Lord, please just get me through this weekend. I don't know why I'm so tense, but I'm afraid if anyone tries to get close to me, I'll shatter into little pieces. Hold me together.*

A weekend of breaking the ice with strangers. Yuck. All day every day, I talked to people. Most days it was fulfilling and fun to be both pastor's wife and church secretary, but lately it was just annoying. Now here I was in an unfamiliar church on a faith-sharing team. It should have been an exciting time spiritually and emotionally, renewing old friendships and making new ones.

What was wrong with me anyway?

Looming deadlines cluttered my mind. But the weariness in my spirit went beyond normal stress. I sat there feeling drained and realized I had no idea why I was there. How could I be an encouragement to anyone else when I was wrestling with demons of my own?

All I wanted that Friday night was to be left alone. But I didn't want to be rude either, so I turned to the gal on my right and found her easy to talk to. We realized we were in the same boat; neither of us knew why we were there. An overload of heavy stuff in her family made her worry that it was the wrong time for her to leave; yet, like me, she'd felt the Holy Spirit's nudge to come.

There was no apparent reason for my funk. My husband was a much-loved pastor, a great spouse, and a loving father for our three grown daughters. We had seven grandchildren and another on the way. We served two great churches. I had dear friends and a fulfilling life and time to enjoy reading and painting. I even dreamed of writing a book about my parents. So many thoughts swirled in my mind and heart as I began that mission weekend.

Saturday morning I found myself seated directly across the room from my new friend. She asked the leader if she could share something and showed us a mustard seed necklace she was wearing. Unexpectedly, I felt my eyes water. Then she took out a container of mustard seeds and began walking around the circle, inviting each of us to choose one. The closer she came, the harder my tears flowed. No one seemed to notice, and I had no idea why I was crying. The unexpected sight of a box of mustard seeds jolted me out of my silent pity-party. What was God trying to do to me?

The rest of the day was a whirl of activity and there was no time to wonder about the puzzling experience until I crawled into bed. Sometime after midnight, the memory was simply there, crisp and clear. I was eight years old and it was my birthday. Someone had given me a mustard seed necklace. Mom found the passage in Luke 17 and showed me how Jesus compared the tiny mustard seed to faith. I was excited. That was the first time I had any idea that Scripture and real life could connect.

I hadn't thought about that necklace for decades. I'd lost it years before. But the mustard seed concept remained a mother/daughter link for many years. When one of us was fearful or discouraged, we only had to mention the mustard seed necklace to get a smile from the other.

How I needed that good memory! I loved Mom but our relationship was very complicated. I dreaded the phone calls when she was drinking. She said and did hurtful things to people I loved. I was often an arrogant and distant daughter. We made real progress in healing our relationship before she died, but until that strange night, I hadn't realized I was still carrying a ton of bitterness and guilt, long after her death.

God was giving me the option of handing it all over to him. So, on a sleepless night in an unfamiliar town, I had a choice. I could curl up with my bitterness and stay stuck, or surrender it to him. It wasn't at all an automatic, "Yes, Lord," moment. Lying there in the dark, I had to face the ugly fact that on some level, I enjoyed my resentment. Over the years, I'd grown way too comfortable with my anger toward Mom. It was so familiar. Letting go of it was scary.

But I did. It was time. I couldn't just ignore those feelings, but I could and did give them to Jesus. He was the only one who could deal with them. They were too tough for me.

Choosing the way of forgiveness was the last piece of a puzzle of healing. Memories of Mom, good ones, paraded through my mind. I could almost smell the delicate scent of her Evening in Paris cologne. I remembered cheering up after a tough algebra test when the scrumptious aroma of her sour cream chocolate cookies greeted me after school. Those memories and others had been buried under the mountain of resentment.

I couldn't wait to see my new friend and tell her I discovered at least one reason we were both there that weekend. I left the little church in that small town a bit weary in body but revitalized in heart and spirit.

LEARNING AGAIN

Throughout the caregiving years, I battled an unforgiving heart more than once. Some days it was directed toward my husband, a nurse, or even myself. It took me a ridiculously long time to catch on to the pattern. Repeatedly, God provided a person, a verse, a song, or his own stubborn love to woo me out of the trap I found myself in.

He always offered me a choice. I could stay furious and wallow in justifying my anger. I could nurse every hurt and every misunderstanding. God wouldn't force me to let go of those reactions. Some days just knowing that the choice was mine made me cringe. Pride, stubbornness, apathy, all tried to block the process. But, oh—the freedom each time I finally yielded to the Father's will.

†·†·†

"With a Special Mercy for Each Hour"

The freedom forgiveness makes possible is always a grace-filled surprise. Each time, it's a breath of fresh air as I receive his miraculous trade. Talk about trading spaces! There really is no comparison. The stupid satisfaction of hanging on to anger can't begin to compare with the delicious delight of letting it go.

If your faith were only the size of a mustard seed, it would be large enough.

Luke 17:6

Prayer: Lord, you alone know the size of this chip on my shoulder. Carrying it around is getting too hard. Move beyond the smallness of my heart with the vastness of your compassion. Teach me again to forgive.

Shirl's Sanity Saver

If forgiveness seems impossible, take heart. That's the stuff Christ specializes in. Invite him to take over. He will, but only if you ask.

CHAPTER 11

When you Need...
HELP
"All My Cares He Fain Would Bear and Cheer Me"

This job is too heavy a burden for you to try to handle all by yourself.
Exodus 18:17b

GOOFY GRANDMA

It was another family get-together at the farm and I was running around downstairs, trying to get food ready and make the living room baby-proof for the littlest ones. It had been a good day and the normal chaos of kids and adults running in and out didn't faze me much. I was tired though, and a bit distracted, wondering how the week was going with Mom and Dad. I heard a soft "Grandma, help..." and then it got louder and there were definitely two voices. Girls. For a minute, I couldn't tell where the sound was coming from but finally I realized it was right over my head. I looked up through the register and there were Shan and Rachel hollering and giggling at the same time. I'd locked them in the bathroom!

Getting them out was easy, but apologizing has taken years. They are both grown now. I'm so grateful they still love their goofy Grandma.

Are there days that being a caregiver makes you feel locked in? Maybe it's time to ask for help.

WHAT IN THE WORLD IS "MINE EBENEZER"?

People ask me all kinds of questions, assuming I have the answers because I'm a minister's wife. Yeah, right! That's about as likely as a caregiver who needs no support. When the Beatles sang "Help!" it seemed cool, but asking for it seldom feels that way. It feels like you're weak, selfish, or not trying hard enough. None of that is true. Everybody, eventually, needs a helping hand.

A few years ago, someone asked me about the line in the hymn, "Come Thou Fount of Every Blessing"[1] with the odd phrase: "Here, I raise mine Ebenezer." I've probably sung that song a bazillion times over the course of our ministry. I must have wondered about it once or twice myself, but apparently, not very seriously. So, since I didn't know and didn't want to admit I didn't know, I did what any normal person would do. I smiled and said, "I'll get back to you on that," and then I went home and looked it up.

The things I learned in my research kept reminding me of a scene in the movie *Mrs. Doubtfire.* As I read the Old Testament account with the term Ebenezer, I pictured Robin Williams in his nanny getup leaping over the tables to perform the Heimlich maneuver on the choking guy, yelling, "Help is on the way!"

The scene I read from the first chapter of 1 Samuel unfolded like a soap opera. In the pilot episode, a priest accuses Hannah of being drunk in church. She's crying her eyes out, dealing not only with her infertility, but also with the fact that her husband, Elkanah, doesn't understand her. In fact, he's clueless about why she's hurting.

But, help is on the way. Maybe you've known a time recently when you felt like no one really understands how you feel or what you're going through, not even those closest to you.

Caregivers are among the most misunderstood people in the world. They can look just fine, putting up a brave front, but be totally falling apart on the inside. I know. I became pretty good at the masquerade myself.

Maybe that's why Hannah's story grabs my heart. I picture her sobbing and I'm cheering, "You, go, girl!" I love the freedom she had to just let her feelings out.

In the next episode, her prayers have been answered and she delivers a healthy baby boy, Samuel. That was great, but before long, the poor kid is in the Israeli foster care system. Well, actually, Hannah's so grateful for the miracle of her son that she surrenders him to the temple. It's an amazing act of love. But can you imagine how the old priest dealt with the endless questions of a toddler? It's enough to make you smile.

Young mothers are among God's most valiant warriors. They, too, are caregivers of the most constant kind. When I was in that season, it was hard, but when I was almost at my breaking point, help was on the way. That's when I gave my life to Christ and he changed everything, starting with me.

Have you ever waited and waited for an answer to prayer and then were dumbfounded at the answer you finally received? That's what happened to Hannah and later, to her son.

Anyway, the bottom line for this story is that Samuel finds himself separated from the only security he's ever known and has to learn how to hear God's voice in a new place. We all have to learn that, sooner or later.

Hannah, meanwhile, went on to have five more children, but every year she traveled back to the temple with a homemade coat for Samuel. It could have been the first example of open adoption. Every time she had to leave him, her heart broke a little, but each time, her faith grew and she knew God was working.

Samuel grew up and learned to hear God's voice, even when it was very hard to swallow. His assignment was to deliver some heavy words to his mentor.

HELP IS ON THE WAY

Now we're finally up to the point in the story about Ebenezer. This was a time of war between the Israelis and the Philistines, even before David and Goliath. It was a mess, but help was on the way.

By this time, Samuel had become a prophet and Eli, in his old age, had to send his sons into battle. The bad news Samuel had been charged with came to pass when those sons were both killed. The Philistines captured the Ark and took it to the temple of their heathen god, Dagon. It looked as if evil had won, but help was on the way. In a scene that not even Steven Spielberg could easily recreate, the Philistines found the statue of their so-called god fallen face down before the Ark. They sat it up again only to return the next morning and find it fallen again, and this time the head and hands were completely broken off. The Philistines' reaction? As our kids today might say, they totally spazzed out. They returned the Ark in a big hurry. In fact, the whole thing was so dramatic that the backslidden, idol-worshipping Israelis repented, and confessed their sins. They geared up to fight the Philistines. It looked like they were hopelessly outnumbered, but help was on the way.

Samuel prayed for his people and they won an amazing victory at a place called Mizpah. That's where he erected a memorial stone and called it Ebenezer (1 Samuel 7:12), which means, "the stone of help." The memorial was an early example of the Rock, the Christ, who is our only real help in any age.

That may seem a long way around the barn to illustrate our universal need for help. If nothing else, the journey of caregiving teaches us that answers often come the long way around. And they rarely come the way we expect.

Have you ever had to tell someone some very bad news? If so, you know how hard that is. There's always a dilemma about doing it gently or just getting it over fast. There's never an easy way to get the job done, but somebody has to do it.

When the bad news landed on us, it seemed like a terrible cosmic joke. We'd watched Dad come to grips with the effects of his stroke: the paralysis and weakness. Now we had to tell him about his lung cancer too. Dick drove all the way up to the hospital in Rochester, NY, to break the news to Dad so I wouldn't have to. I can close my eyes and still see the compassion on Dick's face. It melted my heart, and I fell in love with him all over again.

He talked to Dad man to man, with sensitivity and quiet dignity. The result was that Dad didn't fall apart. He simply decided to take things one day at a time and make the most of the time he had left.

✝·✝·✝

"All My Cares He Fain Would Bear and Cheer Me"

Don't be afraid to admit you need help. You do. It doesn't mean you're weak or inadequate. It just means you're only one person and the needs are huge.

God is our refuge and strength, a tested help in times of trouble.

Psalm 46:1

Prayer: Father, whatever I have to face today or tomorrow, let me realize that help is on the way. You are still in control.

Shirl's Sanity Saver

Face the reality that your ultimate help comes from heaven, but realize that you also need help in the here and now. Call, e-mail, or text someone and ask for one specific thing you need. Do not feel guilty about asking. The ability to help you may just be a blessing to someone else.

CHAPTER 12

When you Need...

HOPE

"He Whose Name Is Counselor and Pow'r"

O Lord, don't hold back your tender mercies from me!
My only hope is in your love and faithfulness.
Psalm 40:11

MISSING AMBER

On my forty-fifth birthday, I'd been home from New York for a couple days and was due to go back the following Tuesday. Mostly, I just wanted to feel sorry for myself because I missed Amber so much. She was all grown up (I kept reminding myself). She and boyfriend, Terry, had graduated from high school and were married the following December. He was in the Navy and they were stationed in Orlando, Florida. I missed her fiercely, and she was on my mind as I read the devotional from *Our Daily Bread*.[1]

My "birthday devotional" included a gift that was a perfect fit for my weary spirit: "When I had lost all hope, I turned my thoughts once more to the Lord... I will never worship anyone but you! For how can I thank you enough for all you have done?" (Jonah 2: 7a, 9a).

Another precious gift came from Dick. My journal records the funny, sweet birthday poem he had written and left for me to find the first thing that morning. He may not be the best poet in the world, but his goofy verses certainly gave my heart the lift it needed. Here are just a couple stanzas for your entertainment:

We started young and dumb
With just a single crumb,
We only wanted some
But look what all has come!

Oh well, no sweat, I'm sure,
Because our love is pure,
A constant, needed lure,
For me, you are the cure.

That wasn't the end of the poetry for my birthday. That night we went to Mary's and she'd written four little poems, each one with a clue to finding the next. It was my own private scavenger hunt and the last verse held a phone number. When I called it, Amber answered in Florida and we were both surprised. She didn't know she'd get to tell me the news. My amazing family had pooled their resources to buy my plane ticket and I was going to Orlando! Looking forward to that trip provided a gift of hope. The next few weeks of caregiving went much better as I thought about the trip. It helped me hang in there on the days that part of me wanted to run away.

Have you been there lately? Discouraged and yearning? Ask God for the gift of hope. Keep your eyes and heart open to a way he might send it. Maybe it'll surprise you too.

FARM MEMORIES

The concept of hope was nurtured in my siblings and me in so many ways as we grew up on that farm in New York. Even in winter, it was beautiful. Tall chestnut trees stood sentinel in front of the house, and the one closest to the driveway was perfect for climbing. There were fields to wander, a huge barn to play in, and enough space for any child to grow big dreams.

Looking back, I'm touched as I realize how often Dad interrupted his endless list of chores to create some extra fun for us. He'd construct tunnels, rooms, and sometimes, whole houses from bales of hay. Often cousins or neighbor kids would join us for the fun.

There were also huge piles of grain to jump in. In fourth grade, a boy name Billy dared me to jump off a beam into one of those piles, promising that if I did, he'd marry me. I did. He didn't.

Dad spent hours putting together blocks of snow for tables and chairs, or forts for us in the winter, and the farm had a swamp that froze over, providing a free ice rink.

Mom did special things that filled our childhood with anticipation, as well. The living room was fairly distant from the kitchen in that big old farmhouse but the sound of a pan sliding across the stove burner carried easily. Carole, John, and I, and sometimes Dad, would look up at each other and grin because we knew what was coming. Soon we heard the welcome sound of popping corn, followed by the aroma of melted butter, and we'd be almost too excited to pay attention to *Father Knows Best*, *The Hit Parade*, or whatever we were watching. Soon Mom came in carrying bowls of popcorn freshly sprinkled with salt. In those days, we had no awareness of cholesterol levels or blood pressure problems. Popcorn was just one of a host of things Mom did to fill our lives with fun.

I always felt proud to drive up the hill to our farm. The fields, lawns, and gardens were all beautifully cared for. Dad usually sang or whistled while he did barn chores, creating a wonderfully safe and happy world to grow up in. He gave us such deep wells of happiness to draw from. Carole, John, and I had no idea, as we grew up in that safe, loving place, that we'd all draw heavily on those memories when things got hard later in life.

The day before I left for college, I climbed to the roof of the house and said a tearful good-bye to the fields from my bird's-eye view. From that lofty perch, I could see the lane behind the barn. I can close my eyes and chuckle at the memory of Hank, our beagle, valiantly helping me bring "the girls" up the lane to the barn. Those cows were actually afraid of that feisty little dog. I remember the day I ran over the fence by the lane. It was the first time I drove the pickup and I was amazed that Dad didn't yell. He just made sure I was OK.

Memories. As I cared for Dad, we'd revisit them. We'd been laughing about the time I drove through that fence on a day that became magical. It started out as a routine round of appointments: a haircut, a stop at the grocery store, and a few other errands. On our way home, I realized Dad was singing along with the radio. Memories of being a little girl, enchanted with a daddy who sang as he milked the cows or drove a tractor or walked down the lane flooded me. He was singing "Moon River"[2] along with the oldies station and the sound was so beautiful to me that I drove past their house and we just enjoyed sharing a few more miles, a few more minutes. I hadn't heard him sing since his stroke.

That day marked a change for both of us. Accepting Christ had changed him from the man who asked me to hide his gun so he couldn't take his own life to the man who added, "Count your blessings, Shirl" to the end of letters from Mom. Hearing him sing was what I needed to realize how deep and real that change was. It gave me hope.

†·†·†

"He Whose Name Is Counselor and Pow'r"

Has God marked a turning point—a day of change—for you? Where has God showed you hope?

> For I know the plans I have for you, says the Lord. They are plans for good and not for evil, to give you a future and a hope.

> Jeremiah 29:11 TLB

Prayer: Lord Jesus, thanks for all the ways hope returns to my heart.

Shirl's Sanity Saver

List the top five things you hope for. By an act of will, trust them to the Father's timing.

CHAPTER 13

When you Need...
JOY
"The Protection of His Child and Treasure"

The joy of the Lord is your strength.
Nehemiah 8:10b

A MOONLIGHT SKATE

The capacity for joy, like for hope, was also sparked on the farm. Memories are such treasures. They help us recapture events long past and hold them close again. I love remembering the winter days when my wanderings took me past the hedgerow, through the last field to the swamp. In the winter, there were none of the pesky mosquitoes that made it so disagreeable the rest of the year. With the freezing temperatures, what had been a muddy, messy bog transformed into my own private sparkling skating rink. It was a place of private joy.

I wasn't a very good skater but it didn't matter down there. I could lace up my skates or just slide around on my boots. As soon as my ankles began to wobble, and they usually did, there was always a tree handy to catch myself on.

One day it was late when I arrived at the swamp, but the skating was better than usual. I skated with a new freedom and sense of fun and before I knew it, the light faded from the sky. I was alone, lost in the darkness, in the middle of a frozen swamp with no possibility of finding a landmark to point me home. Joy skidded to a halt with my skates.

I moved from the knowledge of God as the Father I instinctively wanted to thank and graduated to yelling "Help!" in my spirit, knowing he heard me. I was just a kid. I hadn't yet been to college or become an arrogant religion major who thought she understood everything and had no need of God.

That night, in the dark, in the cold, I knew I needed help. The moon came out, lighting my way home, and the joy that returned was so deep I knew God was in it.

MOM, THE COMEDIENNE

The summer following Dad's stroke, Mom got tired of the gray cloud hovering over the house. She decided it was time to bring some laughter into Dad's life and she used a variety of methods to do it. She started with a series of funny videos after she read that Norman Cousins discovered healing power[1] in laughter. Maybe she took his ideas a little too seriously. Mostly Dad ignored the movies or fell asleep after the first ten minutes. But on the day she put in a Victor Borge tape, she hit pay dirt. First, he chuckled and then as the wacky pianist/comedian grew zanier, our glum Dad laughed aloud. It was the most wonderful sound we'd heard in that house for a long time.

Encouraged by that success, Mom took on a new personality, becoming a bit of a comic herself. She'd give his wheelchair a quick shove, pretending they were racing to see if they could beat yesterday's record. Then she'd do a silly dance, and shake his medicine bottle like a percussion instrument. One night, after that tactic produced half a grin, she turned to me and said, "We're going to make it. He's worth it. I'm a slow learner..."

I told her, "Oh, Mom, I think you're way ahead of us."

And, by God's grace, it was true. Even in the middle of that sad situation, the heavenly Father tucked bits of joy into unexpected moments.

PILLOW NOTES

Those moments of joy repeated several times over the twilight years. One of my favorites occurred the day I heard Dad sing with the radio when we were running errands. I captured the joy in a letter I wrote to him and left on his pillow the day I left to go home for a while.

Dear Dad,

I love you!

Hi again. Now it's Friday morning. I guess I wasn't awake enough to write much last night. But this morning I feel great and I've been sitting here at the table reading about God's love and just soaking it up in this house. His love is everywhere I look. It's in the paintings you've done and the phone list on the wall out in the kitchen, where Mom lovingly fixes meals with those special touches of hers.

And it sure was surrounding us yesterday in our comings and goings. I think maybe it was coming back from Denny's when the radio played, "Moon River" and I noticed you, very quietly, humming along. Then you were singing! Oh Dad, what a beautiful sound that was to my ears and my heart. It was as if God were whispering, "See, don't worry so much about him. I'm still giving him times of joy, even now." I wanted to take that moment and make it last forever.

It's time to write to your darling bride, my lovely Mom, who also amazes me with her strength and faith, even when she's weary. I love it when I can still catch you cuddling. And as Dick and I visit so many people who are living alone, trying to somehow make it, I thank God that you still have each other to lean on and to bring each other joy.

Love,

Shirl

JOY COMES IN THE MORNING

One Sunday in March, I was unwinding from another round of days with Mom and Dad and yet another re-entry process with Dick and the girls when I got home.

After Dick went to bed I indulged in a good cry, releasing the pent up sadness from seeing people I love hurt. Dick was still involved in the long process of painful therapy for his sore shoulder. In New York, the doctor had to re-break Mom's wrist when it was healing the wrong way, and she said it made the original injury on the icy ramp seem easy. I wept for her pain and Dick's, and in sorrow for my own sinful, arrogant attitudes. I was full of resentment toward Mom, stemming from old wounds and I was dragging my feet about letting go of them. As the tears fell, I surrendered this new layer to Christ and then the tears became a gentle cleansing, full of mercy and healing.

That Sunday morning I read this verse: "Oh praise the Lord, for he has listened to my pleadings! He is my strength, my shield from every danger. I trusted him and He helped me. Joy rises in my heart until I burst out in songs of praise to him" (Psalm 28:6-7).

†·†·†

"The Protection of His Child and Treasure"

Weeping is sometimes the first step to surrender. But joy comes with the cleansing, full of mercy and healing.

Weeping may go on all night, but in the morning there is joy.

Psalm 30:5b

Prayer: *Lord Jesus, restore to me the joy of my salvation. I've been moping long enough.*

Shirl's Sanity Saver

Find an old comedy on the movie channel or do some crazy thing just for fun. Laugh at a child or at yourself. Force yourself to smile and then wait for the joy to come.

CHAPTER 14

When you Need...
LOVE
"Is a Charge That on Himself He Laid"

Show me your strong love in wonderful ways.
Psalm 17:7a

LOVE STORIES

There's nothing like a good love story, especially, a true one. Dick's mom loved to tell about falling in love with his dad at a Hopalong Cassidy double-feature movie. Sometimes love at first sight really happens, and lasts. For others, falling in love is more gradual, like the couple who grew up together and one day he looked at her and said, "Wow." Dick's grandmother had a great story like that.

Coming to Christ can also happen softly, little by little, or more powerfully, in a kind of joyful surprise. But, until we come, nothing else really matters much. When we come, it's always because we need his love.

It's love that makes the difference in caregiving. Duty can draw us to the bedside and responsibility might keep us there, but only love can take a situation from a resigned obligation into a place of tender, genuine caring. Without it, the myriad of chores and decisions quickly become things to endure rather than experiences to share.

A NEEDED REMINDER

Some days, Dad was hard to love. He became so angry or ornery or just sullen that I hardly recognized the guy. Mostly, Carole took the brunt of his irritation since she was there the most, and so was the handiest target. It broke my heart because she was our solid rock, always cheerful, and so giving and kind. There was a day when I longed to remember the kind of man Dad used to be and God found a way.

I was sorting papers back in the parsonage in Pennsylvania one dreary afternoon, dreading my next trip to New York. Tucked in a bottom drawer of my desk, I came across two folded pieces of paper with Dad's handwriting. The note was dated September 14, 1965, the day I entered college. That summer, I'd been the one to drive him to the hospital after an accident when baling wire snapped and injured his eye. Curling up with an afghan in my favorite corner chair, I read:

Dear Shirley,

Hi, Honey, how are you doing? First, I get hurt and get everything all goofed up, and then the time goes quickly and it's time for you to leave before I realize it. All the things I wanted to say and all of the good and fatherly advice I was supposed to give, I just couldn't say that day. It suddenly dawned on me that instead of you being the one to be homesick, it was going to be us.

I do want you to know that I love you very, very much and that I am also pretty proud of you. This business of going to college and stuff is all part of growing up I guess, it just has to be done. But I got thinking that even though we all get older, we all are still growing up. Me, because this is the first time I ever had a daughter going to college.

But time marches on and soon Carole and John will be [out of school too] and we'll all grow up a little more.

Bette and I went down to see Dr. Prindle this afternoon and he said the eye was coming very good. He said maybe I could get to work after Saturday. He gave me one of those eye tests where you read the letters and I did real good. Last night was the first night of bowling. I did not bowl but Bette and I went over and just watched for a while.

I don't know if I had two good eyes whether it would improve my writing or not but if you can read this I promise I'll write some more. And if you can find time, don't you forget we like to get letters too. If you forgot anything or need anything write or even telephone. It's not nearly as far as Puerto Rico.

Love you always,

Daddy

A BREATH OF FRESH AIR

The line about Puerto Rico was a reference to a trip my sister had taken. Dad had never seen phone bills like the ones from there, but he didn't really mind. As a high school Junior, Carole had been chosen for a mission study trip to a place she'd wanted to see ever since Frank began spending summers with us. He was a six-year-old boy from the Bronx who came as part of the Herald Tribune Fresh Air program. I can still picture that handsome, adorable little guy, all dressed up in a three-piece suit, running flat out in the parking lot where we'd stopped at the Newark Rose Gardens. We were afraid he was trying to run away, but he was just relishing the freedom of more open space than he'd ever seen before.

Frankie came back summer after summer for years (without the fancy suit), and even spent a couple of Christmases with us. We considered him family. Dad had taken us to New York City to visit Frank's family one year and the stories Mr. Rivera told about Puerto Rico sparked an interest in Carole's heart.

The letter reminded me of the depth of Dad's love, not only for us, but also his willingness to share his heart and home with a young boy from the city. That memory made it easier to overlook the occasional grumpy days he had in the twilight time. His love was still there, stronger than ever. I couldn't let his crankiness make me forget how he gave his love freely, and how much we loved each other.

On days when I'm testy, God looks right through it with eyes of love and sees my hurt. When I let him, he melts my stony heart and teaches me all over again how to let his love flow. And my heart can run free, in the open space of God's acceptance.

LOOKING FOR MR. RIGHT

Before Facebook, Twitter, and MySpace, kids kept up with each other by passing notes in study hall. I remember it well. My friend Linda and I would share earth-shaking news like: "He smiled at me in the hall." Of course, without naming names, each of us knew who "he" was in the other's life, at that moment.

Ah, the great search for "Mr. Right." In Jr. High, we were both a bit shy. By the time we found ourselves at Lycoming College, we were braver.

The Rev. (as I fondly refer to Dick) and I found each other in a philosophy class, and when he called me Mary by mistake in the dining room, I was tickled. I'd always secretly wished my parents had named me Mary. These days, he does many things that tickle me, and some that drive me nuts. But mostly, he still makes me smile.

Being married to this man has taught me so much about love, but I've also learned about love from our grandchildren. May I share a couple of stories that still warm my heart?

RAVEN

Raven was spending the night with us. I tucked her in, and sat on the bed for a few minutes. When she was almost asleep, she whispered, "Can I go downstairs and see Grandpa one more time?"

"No, honey. Go to sleep."

"But, I love him so much."

Before I could think of a snappy comeback, she was snoozing.

RUBY

Ruby had never said a whole sentence to me until the day she said, "I wub you, Gamma." It made my day. What am I talking about? It made my week. Every time I got at all down or discouraged about anything, I just called up that memory and was instantly on top of the world again. Love makes all the difference.

†·†·†

"Is a Charge That on Himself He Laid"

When we long to do something to bless the heart of God, there is no better way than to just say, "I love you, Lord."

Love does no wrong to anyone. That's why it fully satisfies all God's requirements. It is the only law you need.

Romans 13:10

Prayer: Lord Jesus, I've been so lazy in loving, and so wimpy. Your lavish love puts me to shame, yet lifts me up.

Shirl's Sanity Saver

Ask the spirit to show you where your love is lacking. Then open yourself to let his love flow through you.

CHAPTER 15

When you Need...

PATIENCE

"As Your Days, Your Strength Shall Be In Measure"

Be patient with each other,
making allowance for each others' faults because of your love.
Ephesians 4:2 TLB

WHY NOT HOP?

Mrs. Keiper came out in the hall before our session at the parent-teacher conference. She'd been the kindergarten teacher for both Mary and Carrie and now was for Amber. Her grin was a bit wacky as she quipped, "I'm glad to see you and Dick finally had a normal child." Her idea of normal might surprise you.

Mary, from the first kindergarten orientation, had taken charge of the other kids, organizing them into teams. She gave some kitchen duties, some were building with blocks, and others clustered around her in a group looking at books. It's no wonder she spends her days now overseeing childcare centers.

Carrie, on the other hand, had been painfully shy and hadn't spoken much to the other children or to her teacher until January of that first year of school. She hadn't even talked to Santa when he visited their room before Christmas. But once she found her voice, she used it to make friends and today she loves to talk!

So, the first two Leonard girls had been almost too good to be true for a kindergarten teacher. But Amber was neither organized nor quiet nor shy. She was rambunctious, to put it mildly. Never sat still. Never quit talking. Full of fun and a bit of mischief.

Being her mom was a huge blessing, but I remember praying for patience often with her. Our parsonage when she was little was a ranch house with a long hallway and she never walked up or down it. She hopped like a bunny. All the time. I cringe now as I remember my own voice, stressing the second syllable, "Amber, stop hopping, now!"

Why was that such a big deal? What if God had programmed her love of jumping to prepare her for all the hurdles she'd one day clear on the track team? Maybe he was preparing her for the life hurdles she handles now in multiple roles of wife, mother, RN, clinical instructor, graduate student, writer. Sigh. I should have been more patient.

GROWING PAINS

On a chilly February evening at my parents' home in Bristol, New York, I sat propped up in bed, writing in my journal, trying to unwind. An hour before, when I went into his room after Dad called me, he chuckled and said, "Sorry, honey. Just talkin' to myself, dreamin', I guess." I grinned back at him, tucked him in again, and returned to the journal. I wrote:

> *I am so tired and so mad at myself for my impatience with Mom. She is wonderful and is trying so hard, but I find myself wanting to yell, "Hurry up!" or, "Just get out of the way so I can do it." How petty those words look on paper. They are petty. Enlarge my heart, Lord.*

DAD STORIES

One day as we sat at our usual places at the table, Dad started telling me stories.

After a bit, I realized these were stories about his childhood that I hadn't heard before.

I ran back to my suitcase, grabbed my journal, and started taking notes, eager to record at least the highlights.

If you've started that journal I nagged you about in the opening chapters, keep it handy the next time you're with the person you're caring for. Or just keep a pen and paper handy. When they start telling stories, grab the pen, and at least make notes. Better yet, record the stories on tape or CD. Ask questions about their childhood or anything from the past. Ask about school, work, or falling in love. One day you'll be very glad you did.

One of the stories Dad shared that day took place at Lake Wallenpaupack, when he went fishing for small-mouthed bass with his Uncle Bill. That was a memorable trip and there were others. Often, Uncle Bill would motion for Dad, saying "C'mon Sport," or, sometimes, "Hey, Lecky." I'm not sure what those nicknames meant, but remembering them made Dad smile. He talked about the year he traded his trombone for a shotgun after he realized hunting wasn't just fun. It was important because it helped provide food for their big family.

But Dad said that the hardest part of hunting, by himself or with one of his brothers or Uncle Bill, was having the patience to be quiet long enough for the game to appear. Dad hated to wait.

Before his stroke, he complained loud and long about how long it took Mom to shop for groceries. After the stroke, he complained about waiting for a doctor on appointment days or waiting for one of "the girls" when a home health aide would be a little late. If Carole didn't call the minute she got home from work, or if John didn't show up exactly when he said he would, Dad complained. His impatience sometimes irked me. I suppose I thought that since Dad wasn't going anywhere, he had no reason to be in such a tizzy.

Now I realize that with the limitations that stroke and cancer brought to his life, watching the clock was simply one way to deal with the parts of his life he couldn't control. Complaining was at least something to do.

PATIENCE BEYOND THE BIRDS AND BEES

Coming to grips with the reality of both Dad's permanent left-side paralysis and Mom's clinical depression wasn't easy either. Many days, both conditions seemed unreal.

Too often, I had little patience with either of them.

In the early days after Dad came home from rehab, we developed our own routine. Daytimes, when it was nice, I'd wheel him out to the back yard and we talked and watched the seasons change. At night, we awkwardly went through the transfer to the hospital bed in the living room and a sponge bath in that bed. I settled down under the blankets on the couch, just a couple feet away. I had to be able to hear him if he needed anything.

Many days, I had precious little patience with either of my parents or their situations and even less with myself. Everything felt so out of control.

I was soon to learn that both Mom and Dad had learned a lot about patience, just waiting for me to be conceived. One night after supper as we sat at the table lingering over coffee, Dad mentioned, "...those shots I took." When I questioned him, he grinned and said, "You didn't know?"

Then he told me the doctor said they would probably never be able to have children, but there could be a chance if he'd agree to take shots. I'm not sure how often he went but he told me that he tried to time his chores in order to get to the doctor's office when he wasn't too busy. If Doc was in a hurry, the shots hurt, but if he was relaxed, it wasn't so bad. I didn't know if they were B-12 shots or if it was even a real treatment, but the fact was that Dad went through it because they both wanted a child so badly. They wanted me.

I remembered asking Mom the normal kid questions about where I had come from. Mom's answer annoyed me. "I prayed for you," she said. It seemed like such a dumb answer. I might have been three or thirteen; I can't remember. It really doesn't matter. What did matter to my immature heart was that I'd asked an honest question about where I came from and it felt like she was ignoring it. I was humbled and grateful and began to appreciate the accuracy of Mom's answer to me as a child. I knew they had been married for nine years before I was born, but I'd never thought much about it. Indeed her prayers had played a major role in ushering me into this world. They had both practiced patience I knew little of in preparation for my coming.

†·†·†

"As Your Days, Your Strength Shall Be In Measure"

Little by little, God taught me to have more patience with Mom and Dad and even with myself. He is such a gentle Teacher.

Dear brothers, is your life full of difficulties and temptations? Then be happy, for when the way is rough, your patience has a chance to grow. So let it grow, and don't try to squirm out of your problems. For when your patience is finally in full bloom, then you will be ready for anything, strong in character, full and complete.

James 1:2-4

Prayer: Lord Jesus, *you've been so patient with me. Give me a hint about how to be more like you.*

Shirl's Sanity Saver

When you feel the knots of impatience start to bind you up, be still and know that he is God. You are not. Take a deep breath; let that sink in.

CHAPTER **16**

When you Need...
PEACE
"This the Pledge to Me He Made"

He is our peace.
Ephesians 2:14 KJV

FAMILY TIES

Strong family ties can offer needed support in times of caregiving. Growing up, I was sure I was part of the best extended family in the whole world: the Thomas clan. Each aunt, uncle, and cousin had a special place in my heart. Benny, Mom's youngest brother, was still in high school when I was in Jr. High and I loved watching him on the basketball court. He played Chinese checkers with me and was just fun to be around. Aunt Eunie, my all-time favorite piano teacher, directed our kids' choir (reminding us to smile!) and Uncle Dick sang at our wedding. Uncle Charlie and Aunt Sheila were pillars of strength for us as Mom achieved sobriety. Then there were the houses with so many cousins! At both Uncle Bob and Aunt Anne's, and Uncle Jack and Aunt Charlotte's there was always something fun going on. Christmases at Grandma and Grandpa's when we were all there were magic. Grandma's rolls were to die for and her lap was always ready to hold one or more of us. Grandpa would get out his fiddle and Aunt

Charlotte or Aunt Eunie would be at the piano. Life was good as we tapped our toes or danced a jig to "Turkey in the Straw," or "Golden Slippers."

During the twilight time, it seemed that whenever Carole or I needed to step back and catch our breath, Aunt Dorothy appeared. She was Mom's older sister and being with her always gave us the serenity we needed. No matter what was going on, her composure was flawless and we could get a new grip on things just by spending some time with her. How we needed her in those days of caregiving! She'd meet us for breakfast or lunch or just come over, exactly when we needed her. Just spotting her across a parking lot in one of her trademark purple outfits lifted our spirits.

When Dad's stroke happened, Aunt Dorothy's husband, Uncle Charlie, was still alive and what a pair they were! I adored them. My nickname for him was "Uncle Philosopher" and he and I spent hours talking about life and swapping ideas. He told me once, after dealing with depression following a heart episode, that in his experience, the best "psychiatrist" in the world is Jesus the Christ. I had to agree.

As a girl, I spent many summers at their house, and loved every minute. Their huge Roman Catholic church seemed so much more beautiful than our "Plain Jane" First Methodist. Spending time with their three sons was always fun and Dick, the one closest to me in age, became a dear friend. Truthfully, I had quite a crush on him at one point, and when he'd come to our school for a dance, I'd be so proud. He was cute and "with it" and knew the lyrics to every rock and roll song on the radio.

When Uncle Charlie died, I crumbled inside. When my brother, John, came to pick me up for the funeral service, I remember feeling very grateful for his presence. In the car, I started to tell him about how I grieved Uncle Charlie's death and how out of control I felt about Dad's situation. I told him I was tired of being a pastor's wife because people expected me to have all the answers and this situation with Mom and Dad made me feel like I had none. I remember he reached over and just put his hand over mine and I felt such peace.

Watching Aunt Dorothy move through her own period of loss, and experiencing her support to all of us throughout those twilight years, I learned to trust God in deeper, fuller ways than ever before. With the trust came his peace.

On one of my visits to New York after Uncle Charlie's death, Dad was sleeping in his wheelchair at the table. Mom met me in the hallway as I was going to put my bag away. She took me in her arms and said, "There really is a peace that passes understanding."

COUNT YOUR BLESSINGS

God's lessons on peace in those days happened in a variety of ways. One of the most memorable ones was the trip to see Amber in Florida. One night Amber and I sat at her kitchen table and she said, "Your eyes look so sad, Mom," and I burst into tears. All day, thoughts had crowded in. *Store this up. These memories of being with Amber will have to last you a long time.* I tried to push them away. I tried to just enjoy the weather and the break from the rest of my life. It was no use. So I told her what I was thinking and feeling and we hugged, cried, and decided it was time for both of us to learn again about counting our blessings.

Earlier in my visit, a bad storm took the power out. Amber was cutting out contact-paper shapes by candlelight for her preschool class when she began singing the chorus of "Count Your Blessings." Then she told me her memory of the first time I taught her what a blessing was. I couldn't remember it at all. She must have been six or seven and had been visiting her friend, Heather, who lived just up the hill behind our house. I guess she'd been there twice that day already and wanted to go again and I wouldn't let her so she was crying. I told her that both of the times she was there to play had been blessings she should count. Somehow, it helped her.

Hearing Amber tell the story filled me with peace. I could leave her in good hands. God's hands. She knew how to fight with praise.

SPARKLY WATER

Fast forward to the year 2002. Some of the grandchildren and I were enjoying a day at the farm. Memories of both Mom and Dad were never far away.

A soft breeze caressed us as little Michael snuggled against me. We were watching his cousins catch crayfish in the creek. My to-do list swirled in my head. It was long. But Michael didn't feel well, and cuddling him was the only thing I really needed to do right then that mattered.

Pointing to the water, he turned his big brown eyes up to look at me. "How does God make the creek so sparkly, Grandma? Mommy loves it when the water is sparkly." The music of the bubbling stream echoed the soothing sound of God's voice deep within my heart. God was telling me to slow down. I needed to listen. As Michael snuggled against me, I felt a contentment that couldn't be matched by completing any to-do list. It was a holy moment.

✝·✝·✝

"This the Pledge to Me He Made"

Corrie Ten Boom advised: "Don't wrestle; just nestle."[1] That's still great advice!

> **Do you want more and more of God's kindness and peace? Then get to know him better and better.**
>
> **2 Peter 1:2**

Prayer: Forgive me for the times I rush through life, Lord. Thank you for tucking surprises into the nooks and crannies of my days. Help me slow down enough to catch the glimpse of your presence tucked into today, and let me soak up your peace.

Shirl's Sanity Saver

Be still, and know that he is God.

.

CHAPTER 17

When you Need...
PERSPECTIVE
"Help Me Then, In Every Tribulation"

Fix your thoughts on what is true and good and right.
Think about things that are pure and lovely,
and dwell on the fine, good things in others.
Think about all you can praise God for and be glad about.
Philippians 4:8

VIEWING POINTS

Years ago, Dick's mother introduced me to the book, *Mister God, This Is Anna*, by Fynn.[1] We each read that book over and over and enjoyed sharing our thoughts about it. One of the things I remember we both loved was Anna's insight that God has points to view instead of points of view. She arrived at that notion after she and Fynn set up elaborate experiments with mirrors and gyros. For me, it was an introduction to the idea that reality has many faces and that only God sees the whole picture.

Many things make it hard to see the big picture. How about: marriage, parenting, friendship, work stress, and illness? Any of them can make us focus on our own reactions, overlooking the feelings of other people. That's natural, but it's a trap.

The adventure of caregiving was one that often found me battling with my attitudes. The struggle to be fair to Dick, our girls, and my parents all at the same time was sometimes an elusive dream, but I honestly thought I should be able to handle it. All I had to do was learn to switch gears, change hats, juggle roles, pray enough, love enough, and try enough.

If I could have seen then what seems so obvious now, that sometimes you just can't do it all, it would have helped.

If I had only understood that better, I might have been free to just listen to the people I loved instead of constantly feeling like I was supposed to fix everything for everybody. Mom often reminded me that we needed to "let go and let God."

I am still trying to learn that lesson.

FOGGY DRIVE

It was Dad's seventy-seventh birthday. With each milestone and holiday since the stroke, the thought that this could be the last was the unspoken reality. Our daughter, Mary and her daughter, Shantel, picked me up for the drive to New York so we could all help him celebrate. Shan wasn't quite four years old but she loved Grandpa Wes and wanted to go. I was so grateful they were coming. I knew that just seeing them would give Dad a lift.

A bonus for me was that with them there to entertain Dad, Carole and I would actually have a chance to talk to each other, a rare treat in those days. We stayed as long as we could and then headed back to Pennsylvania, leaving later than we'd planned. The trip home was fine until we started over Bloss Mountain, and hit heavy fog. Guilt and relief seesawed in my heart while I thanked God that Mary was driving. I watched her rub her neck, knowing it probably ached from the tension of searching for the edge of the road. We were both so grateful for Shan's unusual quietness. I thought she must be sleeping, but looked back and found her grinning that sweet grin, so much like her great-grandpa's. We were relieved to get to the bottom of the mountain and leave the fog behind.

Finally, I walked in the back door, so glad to be home. Dick, on the other hand, was just upset that I was late. (We had no cell phones in those days.) He and Carrie had tried to wait supper for me since they expected me at six, but Carrie had already had her insulin shot, so she had to eat. I answered him with shortness. Before I left, I had fixed potato salad and had other things ready so they'd be able to eat whenever they were ready. I thought I'd told them that but in the rush to leave, I guess I forgot.

Eventually we all sat, ate, talked, and caught up on what had been happening, and the tensions melted away. There were so many silly little misunderstandings. Once we three realized what life had been like for each other that day, our perspectives were totally different and the fog lifted.

The next day, Carrie gave me a scripture card. It read, "The Lord lifts the fallen, and those bent beneath their loads" (Psalm 145:17). Those words and Carrie's gesture helped give me perspective.

ESCAPE PLAN

Another lesson in perspective still makes me smile, all these years later. Interestingly, it happened the week of Dad's birthday too, his seventy-ninth this time. I'd been home in Pennsylvania a couple days after helping Dad celebrate in New York. Dick was upstairs shaving, getting ready for an Administrative Board meeting. There was a soft knock on the back door and when I opened it, there stood Shan's big brothers, Ryan and Nate, with suitcases. They were not quite nine years old, and their house was just up the road. I ushered them in and joked, "Have you come to live with us?"

In unison they said, "Yeah, Grandma, we ran away."

Their mother's terrible action? She wouldn't let them take a bath before their little sister. I found out later that Shan's hair was full of something sticky so her bath took precedence. "You're weird, boys," I told them with hugs as I scooted them into the living room. I got them busy with something, called their mom, and the boys and I had fun until she got there.

The guys and I had some apple juice then started looking things up in an old set of children's encyclopedias. Ryan thought the meteors were pretty neat. Nate wanted to look at the trucks. I taught them some anger-control tricks, especially one I made up on the spot about counting to ten Grandma's way. You start fast with a rushed, "one-two-three-four," and then, slow down after five and by nine you have to smile. By ten, all the mad would leak out. They liked it. By the time Mary got there they were both ready to give her a big hug.

As silly as that incident was, it made me realize that emotionally I'd run away too many times when I didn't get my way. I pictured God patiently smiling, loving me, and waiting for me to let the bad feelings leak out.

You may feel like no matter what you do, as a spouse, or child or parent or friend, that it's the wrong thing.

It's not.

All you can do is pray for wisdom each day and follow the light you're given for the current situation, and, let it go.

✝·✝·✝

"Help Me Then, In Every Tribulation"

Even those things that feel the most horrendous are only temporary.

Now your attitudes and thoughts must be constantly changing for the better.

Ephesians 4:23

Prayer: Lord, it's hard to know what's really happening to the people I love, and how I should feel or act. Please help me see this from their point of view, and yours.

Shirl's Sanity Saver

Look at the world through a child's eyes. If you don't have a little one in your house, visit a young mother or volunteer in Sunday school. It doesn't matter what you do. Play, talk, or just hang out together. It will do you good.

CHAPTER **18**

When you Need...
SELF-CONTROL
"So to Trust Your Promises, O Lord"

Now your attitudes and thoughts must be
constantly changing for the better.
Ephesians 4:23

NEW BEGINNINGS

There were days during the twilight years when I honestly didn't want to control either my actions or my moods. I felt like I'd earned them. I became skilled at privately considering myself the all-giving, self-sacrificing gal who deserved to vent. Of course, my stupid, petty attitudes were known all too well to God, but for a while, He'd let me rant inside. Eventually, though, it always caught up with me.

During a particularly bad spell, my journal captured this exchange:

Tues. November 5, 1992

Jesus was tired from the long walk in the hot sun and sat wearily beside the well. (John 4:6 TLB)

In your weariness, Lord, you were still filled with compassion for the woman who came thirsting for more than water. In mine, I continually become sullen and a real downer for this family. I need not just forgiveness, but a new strategy.

Wed. November 22, 1992

You are the Lord of new beginnings!

Libby and Dru's toast, on the TV show, "Life Goes On":

"To remembering what matters and forgetting what doesn't."

You can even use a TV show to get your Spirit to speak to me, Lord.

Now there's a song doing it: "Keep pressing on, until the wounds have mended."

Why have Dick and I seemed to be wounding each other lately? I can be unreasonable and touchy. He can be insensitive and stubborn. I get defensive; he gets critical. He thinks I'm too emotional; I think he's cocky. We misjudge each other so often. Yet for nearly a quarter of a century, you've been teaching each of us to look to you for patience with the other. In the ebb and flow of our crazy moods and even crazier situations, we are renewed in love and hope over and over and over again.

I dream of being thinner, sweeter, and easier to get along with. Does he dream? Right now, he's finishing the evening sermon and will soon be on his way down to join me here at the farm. He'll be drained and tired. Why did I have to be such a grouch this afternoon?

Friday was tough. Coming home from New York I stopped at Bath and bought a pretty black nightie. It was a good move. But after the delightfully wonderful loving, I found myself wishing he'd just stay upstairs in the office and let me bustle around in peace. As always on my homecoming days, the hamper and garbage can were both overflowing and I was already so tense about things in New York. I'm not brave enough to just share my thoughts and feelings with him. He'd think me too emotional, too involved. I just raced around, rushing by him as he stood in front of the wall heater, blocking my path until I wanted to scream. Finally, I looked at his face and realized that he wasn't trying to be a pain; he'd just missed me. He'd been both bored and lonely, and he was tense too.

The journal goes on to record thanks for the chances we had to start over each day and of the warmth between us over the next weeks, as we both got better at controlling our moods and sharing our hearts.

A couple years later, my journal recorded a different kind of re-entry from the New York to the Pennsylvania life:

It felt so good to get home and be wrapped in Dick's arms. I let the tears come. He didn't try to give me advice or tell me to "quit hitting my head against a brick wall." He just held me and said he knew this was hard.

MIND GAMES

There was a tiny couplet in the *Daily Bread* in March of 1992 holding advice that both encouraged and convicted me:

SELF-INDULGENCE IS THE LAW OF DEATH;

SELF-DENIAL IS THE LAW OF LIFE.

I wrote this letter to God in my journal that day:

You and I both know that I've been way too self-indulgent, and not just in eating, but in attitudes. How grateful I am that your mercy is new every morning.

Sigh. The struggle with secret eating had been a nagging reality for so long that I was sick of even thinking or praying about it. I rationalized it in all kinds of creative ways.

I deserve this little pleasure. My life revolves around meeting needs for Dick and the girls, and now my parents. So what if I want to lock the bathroom door, sit on the edge of the tub, and gobble pretzels or Oreos, or whatever the current fix is. It's not heroin. What's the big deal?

And so my brain and my spirit did a tug of war and God loved me anyway. Go figure.

REALITY CHECK

One of our biggest challenges came two years later when it was time to face the fact that Dad had to go to a nursing home.

Carole and I both would have taken him into our homes if it had been possible.

It just wasn't. He needed round-the-clock care and neither of our homes was set up for life in a wheelchair. The money our parents had carefully saved had been all but used up in the four years of in-home care. No matter how we crunched the numbers, there was only enough left for a few months. We explored every possible option and finally ended up checking out several nursing homes. It was the last thing we'd ever thought we'd do.

The spring/summer of 1994 when we had to make these decisions, self-control was an elusive thing. Dick was recovering from a painful skin graft on his ear after a skin cancer was removed. He'd dealt with these cancers before. We'd lost count of how many, but this was the first one that needed a graft. Leaving him was torture, but there was an appointment in New York with an eldercare specialist and Carole,

John, and I all felt like we needed some professional advice. Some days I had to fight to control the urge to scream with the frustration of so many needs pulling at me.

Have you been there lately? Go ahead, go outside and yell a minute if it'll help.

LETTING GO

Tuesday June 28, 1994 - Bristol

"So take a new grip with your tired hands, stand firm on your shaky legs..." (Habakkuk 12:12 TLB)

Here I am, back again, and trying to wake up enough to face the challenges of this new day. Its 6:45 a.m., I've been awake since 4:30 when Dad started calling... At 7:30, the day health aide, Lyn, will come early so I can drop off the night health aide, Mabel, on my way to pick up Carole and try to find our way to Monroe Ave, by 9:00. I know I can trust you for all this and to guide us through the house selling stuff.... There's time for a quick breakfast and we're off to meet the eldercare consultant. We sure can use some professional advice. At least, I think we need it.

10:42 p.m.

Only three crying spells today, not bad. Carole had the first one in the office on Monroe Avenue and I had a small one. Then, after John and Carole left, I had a good cry and now, just as I'm ready to sleep... suddenly at the table I felt like I'd fall over if I didn't lie down. Things seem very fuzzy. But I could almost hear Mom whisper, "Let go and let God."

†·†·†

"So to Trust Your Promises, O Lord"

And in the mystery of the Spirit's work, when I let go of trying to control everything, He handed me the gift of a new level of self-control. Amazing.

> But when the Holy Spirit controls our lives, he will produce this kind of fruit in us: love, joy, peace, patience, kindness, goodness, faithfulness, gentleness and self-control.
>
> Galatians 5:22, 23

Prayer: OK, Lord. I admit it. I'm not so good at controlling my moods or my actions or reactions. Please send the Holy Spirit to give me the strength of mind and will needed for this season in my life.

Shirl's Sanity Saver

Make a list of areas you need better self-control. Don't beat yourself up about it. Just face it.

CHAPTER **19**

When you Need...
STRENGTH

"That I Lose Not Faith's Sweet Consolation"

I want to remind you that your strength must come from
the Lord's mighty power within you.
Ephesians 6:10

GRANDMA ERIE

I wish you could have known Dick's Mom. She's one of the major reasons he's so terrific. I wasn't always the most patient and loving daughter-in-law and I'm not proud of that. But early in our marriage, she and I became great friends and we discovered that we shared the same taste in books, music, and people. She listened with an open heart and I could tell her just about anything.

Plus, she was a very fun Grandma! Our girls adored her and they grieve deeply for her still. They called her "Grandma Erie" because that's where she lived. She had an enormous influence on each of them that will remain among their greatest treasures.

Martha Leonard, or "Mum," had a strength of spirit that came from enduring many losses. As a child, her biological father had deserted the family. That loss, none of us knew about for a long time. She had multiple miscarriages and been widowed in her thirties. She raised three children alone, taught school, and became a highly respected and deeply admired woman. But it wasn't until she was nearing her last decade that she hungered for strength of a deeper kind.

I remember the day she and I discovered together the truth of 1 John 5:13, "I have written this to you who believe in the Son of God so that you may know that you have eternal life."

We marveled together that the promise was for us to know, and that we didn't have to wonder, try, or even merely hope about our chances of getting to heaven. It was a promise to lean on totally. It gave her enormous strength for challenges ahead of her that would shake us all.

UNWELCOME NEWS

It was November 17, 1992, when Dick's sister, Mary called. We were surprised to learn Mum had been having trouble with her speech and had experienced short intervals of confusion. The episodes didn't last long so neither of them worried much until that Monday, when for the first time, Mum couldn't read. The doctor said possible causes included a blocked artery, a thyroid problem, or small stroke. Her voice sounded fine on the phone that night, so we were concerned but not alarmed.

What a difference a day makes. Wednesday, November 18, brought a diagnosis of advanced cancer that stunned us. The specialists decided it had probably started in her lungs and spread to her brain. Dick made plans to go to Erie right away and I marveled at how strong he seemed as he handled this new challenge. But I also knew his heart was breaking. He was trying very hard to hide it.

His brother, Mark, flew in from Phoenix and Mum was grateful to have all her children with her. That week the doctors discovered nine tumors in her brain, five of them active. Dick called home and asked me to come and bring the girls. It was the strangest, most memorable Thanksgiving any of us ever spent. Once we all hugged hello and were settled in the living room, our tears came. Mum shook her head, smiled, and said, "Now, I want us to be happy." She eased us into a love-filled conversation that flowed back and forth from small talk and catching up on news to her feelings about the cancer and her thoughts about each of us. After a while, it was clear she'd had enough and she wasn't too subtle about shooing us off to bed. We didn't mind at all. None of us slept much, but we were all just so grateful to be there. Sharing the sorrow with each other made each of us a bit stronger.

TOUGH LOVE

The next weeks were a blur of trips to New York for me and to Erie for Dick, with stabs in between at taking care of our family and our churches. My parents were both in and out of the hospital, and for a while, we wondered who would die first.

In Erie, hospice was called in as Mary, Dick, and Mark did everything in their power to make sure Mum would be able to stay at home until the end. It wasn't easy.

On Sunday, February 7, Dick delivered a meditation for the Communion service that blessed me deeply. It was the true story of his most recent hospital visit with Ken, a parishioner who was in terrible pain but whose first question was, "How's your mother?" Dick told us that he hadn't felt the depth of Christ's love for him like that in a long time, and of how, in effect, Jesus, in his own suffering on the cross, looks at each of us deeply and asks, "How are you?" It was a holy moment. The icy exhaustion of the last few weeks melted in the warm strength of those words.

The following day Dick and I both went to Erie. At 2:30 a.m. Wednesday, February 10, Mum's battle was over. The morning before, while Dick and his sister, Mary, were out, Mum had said to me, "I'll see you in heaven," with the most beautiful smile.

We were all wrecks in those days, worn out with work and grief and things beyond words. And yet, we received power enough to do what needed to be done.

When the Bible tells us that his strength is made perfect in our weakness, that's not just rosy thinking. It's the way it is.

PURE GOLD

A few days later, I wrote in my journal:

Monday Feb. 15, 1993

Jesus told him, "I am the Way—yes, and the Truth and the Life..."
(John 14:6)

It is impossible to describe the impact of Dick's interpretation of this passage on Saturday at the funeral. In over two decades of ministry, it was his finest work. And, his sister, Mary, amazed us all. We knew she was going to read the Christmas letter that Mark had written to Mum. We knew it would be difficult. Mary had never done any public speaking and had always dreaded the moment she'd have to get up in front of people. Only once, as she read through Mark's list of things that he promised would always make him think of Mum (like—a covered bridge, getting a cup of coffee and taking a ride, etc.), did she almost lose it (with the hummingbird I think)... But she went on to finish the letter in a strong, clear voice, and then looked up from the paper and talked from her heart about these last months. She made us all laugh (about the day Mum made her stop to buy shoes for herself and she ended up getting two pairs) and cry (over the day, the last time they'd gone out, when Mum sat in a hard chair in a crummy garage so Mary could get the car's thermostat fixed and be warm when she drove). Mark's part was very good too. He spoke of the respect, love, and gratitude that filled him because of her. He told about the first time he saw Mum hold, rock, and croon to his daughter, Beth and of how, for an instant, it was him she held.

But the treasure of the morning for me came from Dick. His whole message was, echoing the words of his opening poem, "pure gold." He'd worked and prayed long and hard to decide just what to put in and what to leave out. It couldn't have been more perfect.

✝·✝·✝

"That I Lose Not Faith's Sweet Consolation"

Prayer can help you decide what to put in and what to leave out. Ask God to show you how to prioritize the demands on your life.

And your strength shall be renewed day by day like morning dew.

Psalm 110:3b

My health fails; my spirits droop, yet God remains! He is the strength of my heart; he is mine forever.

Psalm 73:26

Prayer: *Lord Jesus, I'm such a mess. I long to be strong for the ones I love, but my body and heart are worn out. Lord, I need you to be strong in me today.*

Shirl's Sanity Saver

Look at a tree. Any tree. Any season. It might be in your yard or in a book. Think about the strength that tree draws from its roots. Look up and read Colossians 2:7.

CHAPTER **20**

When you Need...
TRUTH
"Offered Me within Your Holy Word"

The Lord's promise is sure. He speaks no careless word;
all he says is purest truth, like silver seven times refined.
Psalm 12:6

FACE THE MUSIC

We learn early and well how to avoid telling the truth, even to ourselves. Little kids become good at blaming each other or the dog for every mess they get themselves into. Big kids perfect the art of making excuses. By our teens and young adult years, most of us are experts at justifying our faults and weaknesses.

It was the centennial celebration of Wallis Run United Methodist Church. I was sitting between Dick and Raven, the youngest of our granddaughters at the time. She snuggled against me, happy to be with Grandma and Grandpa for the afternoon.

With Raven cuddled at my side, it was nice to let my mind drift back to what life was like when we served Wallis Run church three decades before. I was pregnant then with Raven's mom, Amber. It didn't seem possible that so many years had passed.

Assuming Dick and I would both speak, I planned my wise, witty speech in my head. When we'd moved into a house in the community, Dick had said, "There's a little Methodist Church just two doors down the road and if you think you want to go and take the girls, fine. Just don't expect me to go with you."

That story would certainly glorify God. I imagined the congregation thinking, *Just look what God's done in their lives since then.* Not only had Dick started going to that little church, he'd entered the ministry there and had gone on to become the assistant to the pastor, preaching each week in at least two of the five churches. Since that time, we'd served a total of sixteen churches and a parade of men and women had gone into ministries of their own under Dick's mentoring.

Then the pastor called Dick to come and say a few words—not me, just Dick. The things he shared were amazing. They were much better than my prepared speech.

Suddenly I realized that God had taken my opportunity away because my heart was all wrong. Under the "give God the glory" motive was my real hidden agenda. I wanted them to think, *Wow—Didn't Shirley have great faith! She must have been quite the prayer warrior.* As I sat there cuddling Raven, I thanked God for loving me enough to show me the truth of my pettiness and pride.

The truth is, Dick may have come to Christ a bit later than I did, but once he did, he poured himself totally into the relationship. He is the most Christ-like person I know. He's had to be, to put up with moody me. His walk with the Lord makes me humble and very grateful to be part of his life.

Facing up to the truth of who we are and how we really think and feel isn't easy. Yet, there is such freedom in it. Jesus wasn't kidding when he said, "You will know the truth and the truth will set you free" (John 8:32).

He knows all about hard realities.

NIGHTMARE DAYS

The hard realities of Dick's mother's death and funeral in February 1993, were a preparation for what was coming all too soon in New York.

Mom called on Tuesday, March 9, to say the forecast looked bad, and I shouldn't worry if I couldn't make it. I was supposed to take her to a doctor's appointment because Carole had to go to the hospital herself for an MRI. I talked to Dad and he sounded overwhelmed and somewhat lost.

Dick and I talked it over and decided I should try to get there before the snow got too bad. Telephone calls from the home health aides had been telling us it was getting harder and harder for them to handle Mom's "craziness" and take care of Dad too. When I arrived, I could see they weren't exaggerating. I couldn't believe how much things with Mom had changed since my last trip, two weeks before. She had been hiding Dad's meds, refusing to use her nebulizer, and becoming more and more disconnected from reality.

LAST LULLABY

Mom's "monster within" grew steadily more unpredictable. She was admitted to the hospital two days after I arrived. Her blood gas numbers were awful and her level of confusion and aggression scared us all. She pulled out her IVs, so the nurses inserted a heparin lock and wrapped it with adhesive tape. She got it soaked on purpose in the bathroom. She pulled off a whole roll of toilet paper and splashed water everywhere before I could get to her. This woman who had been weak and feeble now developed an alarming strength. I was so grateful to John when he went to the other side of the bed and stroked her forehead. It calmed her down enough so she quit screaming and even ate a few bites of her sandwich and all her ice cream. But then I let my guard down and wasn't smart enough to take off my watch. She grabbed it and pulled with an iron grip. One nurse said that adrenalin levels are elevated in emphysema patients and explained that Mom really wasn't responsible for her actions at that point. Carole finally had to come help me pry her fingers open. An hour earlier, I had to pry Mom's fingers from Carole's hand.

Mom hurt a nurse badly with her fingernails and they had to up the dose for her tranquilizers. Once she was sleeping deeply, I went to the nurses' station and asked for nail clippers. As I cut her nails, I wanted to weep. It felt like cutting long hair on a beautiful girl. I thought that if she ever snapped out of this, she'd be horrified. She always took such beautiful care of her nails.

Her doctor said she was in classic end-stage emphysema and that the CO_2 build- up was causing the confusion. On the up side, he guessed that it should bring a quick, painless death.

Then her respiratory therapist came and said he'd seen her come back from worse episodes than this one and she might go on for quite a while yet. I was screaming inside, desperate to know which of them to believe.

It was so hard to know what to do. Part of me wanted to jump in the car, get home to Dick, and have some time with him before he had to go back to Erie. There was so much paper work still needing attention after his mom's death and Mary needed his help. I missed him so much. I imagined how nice it would be to lean into his strength. But he wasn't in New York, so I poured my thoughts into my journal:

Tues. March 16, 1993

Still here. After I got Dad in bed, I went into the laundry room to throw his clothes in the washer. There was a pile of clean towels on the top and I leaned on them, cried for a while, and felt your strong comfort. She has pneumonia. Dr. S. said if it were his Mom, he'd stay, so I'm here until Friday. Then, if nothing's changed, I'll go home for the weekend.

(Journal 3/16 continued)

Just got off the phone again. Whew. When Dick finally agreed that I'm not "wasting my time" here, I felt such a relief. On last night's call, when he was acting as if we should put Dad in a nursing home, it felt like he'd kicked me in the stomach. But I know it's out of love and concern for me. I was such a wreck, and hearing his voice was what I needed.

Today Mom was calmer, far from normal, but calmer. They upped her oxygen to five and doubled her tranquilizer. The doctor said morphine's the next step. I sang to her, "I Love You, a Bushel and a Peck," to try to get her off the "comedy" track. She started to sing but was hollering so loud. I switched to "Count Your Blessings" and she quieted down, sang along with the chorus, and went to sleep.

In a rare lucid moment, Mom had told me what color she wanted to wear for her funeral and recited half of the Lord's Prayer. I left the hospital wondering if I'd ever see her again.

By that time, the "Blizzard of '93," was on the way, so traveling home to Pennsylvania wasn't an option. With the big storm coming, someone had to stay with Dad and I was grateful it could be me. We had kerosene heaters, bottled water and candles, but amazingly, never needed them. The power stayed on but the roads were closed. Nearly fifty inches of snow fell, with winds of sixty miles per hour. Dad and I were snowed-in at their house for six days. Our time together was precious, even with the curtain of sadness surrounding us. We enjoyed *Lawrence Welk* and other favorite shows and watched the snow pile up to unbelievable levels.

When the plows finally cleared the roads and the home health aides could come stay with Dad, I went back to the hospital. Things were even worse than they'd been six days earlier. I fell apart. Mom bit her tongue, thumb, lips, and a nurse's glove. Her seizures were terrible. She screamed, "It hurts." I lost it completely when she pushed her foot through the bed rails and it took three of us to get her unstuck. Plus, they were still doing blood gases and for some reason, were doing finger pricks for diabetes, a condition she'd never had, and one that wouldn't have mattered at that point any way. When I challenged them, they admitted it wasn't on her chart but was "just routine." I said, "Not anymore it isn't."

I remember marching to the phone in the hall, not trusting myself to ask at the nurses' station. I called her doctor in the middle of his office hours. I insisted that he order comfort measures to start immediately. I said, "It's both cruel and pointless to let her go all night like this."

To my amazement and great relief, he agreed. I thanked God for giving me the freedom to be a loud, obnoxious daughter right then. The truth was that it was time to yell. He called in the order and they started the morphine.

Soon after I got back to Dad's house, John called from the hospital. He said that right after the second shot of morphine, the frown lines in Mom's forehead eased up and the shaking went way down. I wept with relief, splashed cold water on my face, and went in to talk to Dad. He decided he didn't want to go see her. I turned off the TV and we had a good talk and cried together.

He wanted to remember her the way she used to be.

I wrote in my journal: *"Me too. This is a nightmare."*

She died just before 4 a.m. on Thursday, March 18, without me there, and that hurt. But the solid truth in Ecclesiastes 3:3 eased the pain. I thanked God for the Word's recorded reality: there really is a right time to die. I was so grateful to be home with Dad that morning and we held each other and shared our grief and our relief that her suffering was over.

✝·✝·✝

"Offered Me within Your Holy Word"

Facing the truth of sickness and death is not much easier than facing the truth of our sinfulness. Whatever it is you need to face today, you don't have to do it alone.

For he loves us very dearly and His truth endures.

Psalm 117:2

Prayer: Lord, there are so many things that confuse me and there is so much I don't understand. I'm counting on the fact that you not only know but you are the Truth.

Shirl's Sanity Saver

Call someone you trust to tell you the truth.

CHAPTER **21**

When you Need...
UNDERSTANDING
"Help Me, Lord, When Toil and Trouble Meeting"

This plan of mine is not what you would work out, neither are my thoughts the same as yours! For just as the heavens are higher than the earth, so are my ways higher than yours and my thoughts than yours.
Isaiah 55: 8-9

FAMILY RELATIONSHIPS

When we were small, all Carole and I did was fight. It seems so dumb now. I have no memory of what we fought about but I know that sometime between when I got married and when she did, we stopped being enemies and became friends.

And then we became, sisters, in more ways than one. Carole and I had been out visiting friends. When we drove back to our parents' farm on the top of the hill, we both knew it was time. I was a new Christian myself and had no idea what I was doing, but the Holy Spirit was in the car, and before we went into the house, we prayed and Carole gave her life to Christ. A year or so before that, my brother had taken me to that Lutheran Church in Canandaigua where I had accepted Jesus.

I'm glad Carole and I stopped fighting. I'm glad God didn't give up on me, or her. When we shared the care of our parents, I learned to love and admire her even more deeply.

Families can be hard to understand. Siblings may have experienced the same events very differently. Challenges of caregiving multiply those differences. No family is perfect. Some people rise to the occasion and pitch in easily (or so it seems). Others care as much, but are so scared that they do nothing.

I don't know how your family deals with stuff. But I urge you to talk things out. Work together where you can. Fill in gaps. Ask for help. Don't expect everyone to feel things the same way you do, or to know how you feel or what you need, unless you tell them. Somehow, the stress of caregiving often makes us forget that the others around us aren't mind readers. What's obvious to you might not be to someone else. And, remember, no matter what, the gift of family is priceless.

HOME HEALTH TEAM

After Mom died, Dad stayed in the house with help from his kids and a team of aides who filled in when we couldn't be there. Home health aides[1] are often given a bad rap. There are a few dishonest or unfit ones and they make it rough for the good ones. A chart on the wall let Dad and the rest of us know who was supposed to be there when. Carole and I had to be careful not to double-schedule or assume one of us would be there without checking. We had some remarkable help. Mabel was the overnight gal who made it possible for me to actually get a little sleep. Lyn was there daytimes and grew to love Dad so much that she spoiled him and that did us all good. Helen was fun, strong, and wise and Karen was giving and easygoing. There were lots of others but they didn't stay as long. Mabel, Karen, Helen, and Lyn became like family and their understanding not only of Dad's needs, but also of what Carole, John, and I felt and needed was such a gift.

I have a picture in my office of Dad in his wheelchair with balloons. His back is to the camera, but I can see his grin in my mind. He's holding the long streamer on a balloon, one of several brightly colored ones "the girls" hung from the ceiling. The curly hanging ribbons remind me of how those girls helped us celebrate Dad's birthday that year. They understood how badly we all needed spots of joy and color in that bleak season.

REALITY CHECK

We wanted so much for Dad to be able to stay in his own home until he died. It just wasn't to be. Eventually he grew so weak, it took two of us to do the transfers from the bedside commode to the bed or the bed to the wheelchair. Financially and physically, we realized our time was running out. The search for a care facility had to begin. Yuck. How we hated that.

Dad's own understanding made it OK. He helped pick out Conesus Lake Nursing Home, where he spent the final months of his life.

The last page of the home-care log we kept to track Dad's condition, medication changes, etc. was from Lyn. Dad called her "Blondie." She wrote, "Wes seems to be handling everything like a champ and that's just exactly what I thought he'd do. The things I've learned from this man are priceless. He has more love and understanding and acceptance than any hundred people put together do. His family is very lucky to have him as their dad and male role model. Thanks for sharing him with me."

She understood how much we all needed to be lifted up at that moment and her words did exactly that.

SALLY LUNN BREAD

I felt like an idiot. There I was, crying, in the middle of the kitchen of the restaurant where Mom had worked for decades, almost nine years after her death. I had pulled into their parking lot on a whim, after leaving my sister's house. It felt good to be in Bloomfield, New York, to be home, to spend time with Carole. Our time together is never long enough. I felt a strong pull to go to the Holloway House[2] even though I wasn't dressed up, and it was a dress-up kind of restaurant.

I pulled into the back parking lot where I'd dropped Mom off for work so many days and picked her up so many nights. I sat there in the car for a long time. The ivy-covered walls had changed very little even after so many years. Entering through the back door of the kitchen, the years rolled away.

The surge of emotion surprised me. It took a bit of courage to tell the cook that I just wanted to buy some Sally Lunn bread.[3] She gave me a strange look and said she had to ask the hostess, the position Mom held for such a long time.

Before the cook returned, a lovely older woman entered and I felt my eyes grow misty. She had to be the owner. "Could you be Mrs. Wayne?" I asked. She was so gracious when I introduced myself as Betty Ford's daughter.

She told me that some of the waitresses had been looking at pictures from the 1958 book recently and there were many of Mom. I would have been eleven. She worked there all through my school and college years. I remembered Mom's pretty dresses, the seating charts spread out on our dining room table, and, the Sally Lunn bread. It was my favorite of all their specialties. Some weeks, she'd bring a half a loaf or so home and it would be a real treat.

Memories of Mom and Rita (another hostess), of Muriel, Jane, Mrs. Talent, Vera, and Bertha Day—the waitresses and cooks that worked with Mom—flooded me and I was helpless to stop the tears. As I drove away, I listened to a CD of Irish hymns and they were a lovely backdrop for my unexpected weeping. It was a holy time. I wondered how people ever work their way through the process of grief-work without the luxury of three-hour car rides.

I felt enormously blessed by those twin gifts of privacy and time. Maybe the greatest blessing was the discovery that I really did miss Mom. I realized that my longing for her was a result of the healing work of the Holy Spirit.

And I felt blessed by the Sally Lunn bread. Dick wasn't home when I arrived, and as I savored each bite of the first slice, I was amazed. It was every bit as wonderful as I remembered. It had probably been close to thirty years since I'd enjoyed that taste. I had some the next morning, toasted. Bliss!

I shared the rest of the loaf with our daughters when we got together for Labor Day at the farm. Mary and Amber both said that the taste reminded them instantly of Grandma. Carrie thanked me for sharing it. What a blessing that was for my heart. Several weeks later, Carrie and I were on our way to a Wayne Watson concert when we talked about it again. I knew from her words that she really understood how much the whole bread episode had meant to me.

WORLD COMMUNION

I was thinking about all of that on a day Dick was preparing his meditation for World Communion services. The bread we share at Communion isn't the Sally Lunn kind. It is something infinitely more precious. We take comfort in this, God's covenant to love, care for and understand us. If there are days when the wonder of his presence bring me to tears, I won't feel like an idiot. Not even a little.

†·†·†

"Help Me, Lord, When Toil and Trouble Meeting"

Each trouble you've endured has been seen and felt by the Father. He gets it when no one else does. When no one else really understands how you feel or why you feel that way, he knows.

> …and he has showered down upon us the richness of his grace—for how well he understands us and knows what is best for us at all times.

Ephesians 1:8

Prayer: *Father, today I don't understand much of anything. I'm tired and grouchy and part of me wants to forget I'm a caregiver. Thanks, Lord, for understanding.*

Shirl's Sanity Saver

You need a break. Set aside at least fifteen minutes to do something easy that will relax your weary brain. Don't even try to understand anything. Trust that God has enough understanding right now for both of you.

CHAPTER 22

When you Need...
VISION
"E'er to Take, as from a Father's Hand"

Slowly, steadily, surely, the time approaches when the vision will be fulfilled. If it seems slow, do not despair, for these things will surely come to pass. Just be patient! They will not be overdue a single day!
Habakkuk 2:3b

THE BARN

On that bright fall Sunday morning, there was no time to read my sister's e-mail before church, so I printed it out and tucked it in my Bible. We have three worship services each Sunday, and it wasn't until the last one that I noticed the e-mail waiting in 1 Chronicles. Carole's news? Dad's barn had finally come down.

The barn was the place we played in the hay forts Dad made. It was the place I earned my Brownie badge for agriculture when I helped Dad do chores. It was where I'd go to look for Dad when Mom sent me with a message or a snack. As soon as I entered, the good smells of grain and hay were there and I'd find him by following the sound of his singing. Sometimes he was whistling, which was even more beautiful.

Carole got hurt in that barn when she was little. Actually, I guess the accident happened in the silo, hooked to the barn with a feeding chute. Dad was forking silage and didn't realize she was running around in there until the pitchfork caught her leg. I don't remember how badly she was hurt, but I remember feeling sorry for Dad because he felt so bad about the accident. He loved us so fiercely, so completely.

The farm had been sold several years before Dad's stroke and I'd lived in Pennsylvania for forty years. Lots of time and distance stood between that old barn and me. Even so, the news in Carole's e-mail made me cry. That was annoying. We were in the middle of church and I was in my usual pastor's wife second-from-the-front pew. Paranoid as it sounds now, I was sure people noticed me crying. We still had to sing the last hymn. The altar hymn. The time when people are invited to come pray for whatever they need. A holy time.

I didn't intend to go to the altar, but there I was, kneeling, feeling silly, thanking God for the gift of that old barn and what it had meant to me. It felt like the perfect way to grieve and I rose from my knees wrapped in the arms of the Comforter. It felt good.

NEW VIEW

Carole wrote that as sad as it was to see the barn reduced to a pile of lumber, she could tell that once the mess was cleaned up, the view from the house would be amazing.

There are times in our lives when God needs to clear away some old ideas, feelings, and attitudes so that we can see clearly what really matters. For too many years, I silently resented Dick because he didn't treat me like a princess the way Dad did when I was little. Poor Dick.

In the early years, I cried over every hurt feeling and didn't have a clue about how to tell him what I needed. He is an incredibly kind and supportive husband. I didn't understand that very well until the twilight years.

In the years Mom and Dad were sick, the Lord had to rid me of idolizing my father and of blaming Mom for every bad attitude I'd ever had. And blaming my mother for my weaknesses was a lot easier than owning up to them and turning the mess over to the Master. How much time I wasted with my inner pity-parties, wallowing in resentments.

Maybe you need a new vision about how to react to life or people. I sure did. How full of grace is the God who created mustard seeds, gravity, and men who build barns that will eventually turn to dust.

MARY'S SONG

Our daughter Mary helped me so many times as I transitioned from Pennsylvania to New York and back. Today she is a busy childcare center coordinator, and a pastor's wife herself, but she was never too busy for a visit as I drove between my home and Mom and Dad's. I'd stop on my way and she'd make tea. She'd listen, and we'd pray. I could cry, vent, feel better, and be ready to do it all again in a few days. These days, Mary and her husband, Mike, help me see how big God's love, comfort, and strength really are.

I always think of the hymn, "Be Thou My Vision,"[1] when I think of Mary. Through the years, she and I have harmonized on that hymn (which is Dick's favorite) in many church services. My own inner vision became cloudy for a while when I hurt my back helping Dad, and the doctor advised me to take a few weeks off to let it heal.

Mary took my place. Before she'd gone into education, she had some training in a nursing home and felt competent to give the personal care her Grandpa would need. Dad loved having her there. When I finally came back, he raved so much about how great Mary was, I almost said, "What am I, chopped liver?"

Mary remembers that, as much as she'd loved and enjoyed time with Grandpa before, those weeks taking care of him were a treasure because they connected on a completely new level. He appreciated every little thing she did for him and they had good talks over some of his favorite TV shows, like *Murder She Wrote* and *Matlock*. There was sweetness and vulnerability about him; their time together held fun and tenderness and she was grateful for it. Mary gained a whole new vision of who her grandpa really was and felt like he could finally see who she'd become as an adult.

TO SEE BEYOND

Dad seldom was angry before the stroke, but I do remember how mad he was one time when Dick took Mary and Carrie up on the barn roof. They were little, but Dick was right there with them and made sure they were OK. He thought they needed an adventure; Dad just thought it was stupid.

I remember Mary's eyes sparkling when they came down. "Mommy, you should have come up with us. You can see to forever from up there."

Only God can truly see "to forever," but in His great mercy, he gives us glimpses now and then.

Sometimes when Dad nodded off in his wheelchair, he'd flip his hand down with a particular repeated motion. It looked familiar but puzzled me.

"He's fishing," John said, and we both smiled, watching Dad dream of that perfect catch still lurking in the deep water

I have visions of my own these days. I long for my children, grandchildren, and great-grandchildren to experience lives full of love, joy, and faith. I want Ry, Nate, and Shan to remember the silly time all of us (and the dog!) were squeezed under the bottom bunk and we had "no worries." I hope all of them will be able to look back and remember my "Lucy the Ladybug" stories. I hope they smile and dream their own dreams and catch a vision of God's amazing, personal love for each one of them.

VISION OF A SPECIAL SPOT

In the middle of August 1994, Carole and I were at Dad's house. She was sitting at the desk, writing checks, trying to juggle the small balance in his account with the payroll for the aides and other bills that had piled up.

We knew we had to make a decision soon about a nursing home. Dad agreed, but thought there was no hurry. We hugged, prayed, and thanked God ahead of time, through tears, for the vision he'd given us of a spot waiting for Dad. We didn't know if it would be in Newark, Avon, Canandaigua, Conesus, or Heaven. We only knew that God knew and that was enough.

†·†·†

"E'er to Take, as from a Father's Hand"

While caregiving, it's easy to lose your vision. Take time to smile and dream your own dreams. Catch a vision of God's amazing, personal love for you.

After I have poured out my rains again, I will pour out my Spirit upon all of you! Your sons and daughters will prophesy; your old men will dream dreams, and your young men see visions.

Joel 2:28

Prayer: Lord, become my vision. You are already Lord of my heart; turn all my dreams and imaginations to you.

Shirl's Sanity Saver

Dare to dream.

CHAPTER **23**

When you Need...
WISDOM
"One by One, the Days, the Moments Fleeting"

I will bless the Lord who counsels me; he gives me wisdom in the night.
Psalm 15:7

DAD'S WISDOM

Unless I read it myself in my own writing in my own journals, I would never believe this stuff. It seems so wild looking back at all the things we were juggling during the twilight years.

Each daughter went through hard places during that time, and when I read the stories of parishioners who needed us, I'm floored. We fumbled around for God's wisdom, especially, in the closing chapters of the story. Dad needed round-the-clock care and when the money was running dangerously low, we knew we had no choice but to sell his house to pay for the residential care he needed. We thought Dad's house was sold several times, but one deal after another fell through. It was tough not to panic.

One of the facilities we'd considered had a bed available but they needed more money up front than we had. Carole and Jim were packing to take their daughter, Jeannine to college. My beloved Dick was facing more surgery. There were so many times when Carole and I felt like we were following the "cloud by day and the flame by night" like the Israelites, being led by God one step at a time.

Carole called me in Pennsylvania on Thursday, Aug. 25, 1994, to tell me about one of God's amazing answers to our prayers for wisdom. She was on a shopping trip with her son, Zeke, and when they got home, Dad's care provider, Lyn, called. She and Dad were out for a ride and he wanted to see the extended care unit in Canandaigua, so they went. Afterward, he wanted to go on and check out the nursing home in Conesus. He wondered if Carole could meet them there. She did. As Carole, Lyn, and Dad toured the facility, Dad seemed to recognize someone. He thought it was our daughter, Mary. Susan, the aide he saw, did look very much like Mary and, when Dad became a resident, Susan took a special interest in him. They became good friends.

The decision was made. Conesus Lake Nursing Home would become the final stop on this journey and Dad was wise enough to know we needed his help to take this hard step.

A few days after Dad moved into Conesus, I penned these words in my journal:

The image of Dad in his new bed, looking so completely relaxed, comfortable, and cozy keeps dancing in my head. I think of how Carole and I prayed together last month, thanking you ahead of time for the bed you were finding for him, when we didn't know where it would be.

How grateful we were that when we needed wisdom to make decisions for our earthly dad, our heavenly Father supplied it, one step at a time.

MOM'S SENSE

How many times when I was little did I hear Mom say, "Betcha twenty cents"? Her eyes would be twinkling and there would be a chuckle in her voice and for a minute, I'd forget to be a smart aleck kid. If I forgot myself entirely, I even chuckled along with her. That silly phrase wasn't especially articulate or cultured, but it was fun. It wasn't until I was in college that I found out she missed being salutatorian of her class by a single grade point. I never considered her either especially dumb or especially smart. I guess I never really thought much about it one way or the other.

Looking back I can see layers of wisdom in many of the things she said and did. She was wise enough to tell me over and over again to *"Let go and let God."* She was on the ball enough to teach me by example that God is color-blind, at a time when the world didn't seem to be so. She was astute enough not to offer too much advice as she watched me struggle with parenting. The only parenting counsel she gave me was something that truly did help. She'd found it in a magazine and passed it along to me on a day I needed to hear it: "Never take anything a teenager says personally."

Mom loved God, her family, and her friends, in that order. She wasn't a perfect mother. I was far from a perfect daughter. But I am grateful for the wise lessons she taught me.

Is there somebody in your life you're especially thankful for today? How about letting them know. It'll mean a lot to them, I think. In fact, even though Methodists aren't supposed to gamble, I'll betcha twenty cents.

TRUE GRIT

I've been thinking about one of Catherine Marshall's bits of wisdom. She's probably my all-time favorite author. If you've never read her or if it's been awhile, I invite you to treat yourself to something special. Go to the library or bookshop or go online and look her up. You won't regret it.

Anyway, as I thought about all the times I enjoyed sharing one of her books with my mom or Dick's, I remembered something I hadn't thought about in ages. Introducing one of her books, Marshall used a memorable analogy. She said that she could finally write about a particular season in her life now that "her colts were across the stream."[1]

You may be currently in or anticipating a season of caring that has you full of questions that you've never faced before. Your "colts" may be older than you are but right now, they are swimming against the current. The dam is about to break. Maybe your mom's falls have become more serious. Perhaps your dad's memory lapses aren't anything you can joke about any more. Sometimes we enter the realm of caregiving little by little. Or maybe, a crisis lands us there with a thump and precious little warning. It can be a very frightening place and time.

The struggle to maintain your parents' dignity and their safety can become a formidable task that can scare the daylights out of even the strongest among us. I cannot claim to be the greatest expert on this, but I can honestly tell you that I know where you can go to find wisdom.

It's not with Dorothy and her trio of characters on a yellow brick road. It's not in a bottle, a pill, an affair, nor from a psychic. My answer may seem simplistic, but it's the only one that I've found that works.

It's Jesus. No kidding. Just typing his name makes me recall the almost tangible feeling of new grit replacing the spaghetti in my spine, and the clearer thinking replacing the straw in my brain.

There were days when I went to Christ, terrified that I was letting everyone in my life down, including him. He never failed to lift me up, even when some of the ways he did it felt harsh or when he seemed to take way too long.

It takes wisdom to juggle the needs of children, spouses, jobs, and parents all at the same time. I was often frightened that if I stayed in New York too long, the girls would suffer, and, of course, at times they did. So did Dick; so did I. But we all survived and today they're grown and face their own juggling acts with grace. Generally, they each do it with a better grip on sanity than I felt at the time.

†·†·†

"One by One, the Days, the Moments Fleeting"

When you need wisdom to make caregiving or even personal decisions, turn to your heavenly Father. He will supply your needs, one step at a time.

> …the wisdom that comes from heaven is first of all pure and full of quiet gentleness. Then it is peace-loving and courteous.

It allows discussion and is willing to yield to others; if is full of mercy and good deeds. It is wholehearted and straightforward and sincere.

James 3: 17

Prayer: *Ah, Lord, how I need your insight for the days ahead. I am clueless about the best way to handle things, even my own heart. Give me a hint, Lord. Replace my foolishness with your wisdom.*

Shirl's Sanity Saver

Read a verse or two from one of the "books of wisdom" each day for a month. Let them speak to your heart. These books include Job, Psalms, Proverbs, Ecclesiastes, and Song of Solomon.

CHAPTER 24

When you Need...

WONDER

"Till I Reach the Promised Land"

Christ came with this new agreement so that all who are invited may come and have forever all the wonders God has promised them.
Hebrews 9: 15a

REBIRTH OF WONDER

"I am waiting for the rebirth of wonder," said the young pastor. It was the opening line of a sermon he was delivering at an ecumenical Lenten service the year I turned nineteen. That was 1963. I don't remember his name, how he looked, or anything else about him. He wasn't our minister. His pulpit was in the Congregational Church across the park from our First Methodist in East Bloomfield, New York. This community-wide service was in the Episcopal Church down the street and I have no memory of what the sanctuary looked like. But I have never forgotten that opening sentence or the inner journey it began in my heart. It changed my life.

At nineteen, I was an arrogant religion major who had outgrown her faith, or so I thought. I went to college looking for the meaning in life and even when I switched from psychology to sociology, and finally settled on a double major in philosophy and religion, the answers refused to come. I was jaded and bored with Biblical studies and explorations of World Religions.

I was home on spring break and the last thing on my mind was going to church. How could I say no to my little sister, though? She invited me to go and I didn't have the energy or the heart to explain to her how irrelevant formal religion really was. She might as well find it out on her own, like I did. I went along to humor her, not expecting to get much out of it.

Then he hit me with that line about wonder. It felt like I'd been jolted out of a long half-sleep. Maybe I'd been bored with the normal churchy words, but wonder was something I did know about, and it was something I missed very much.

The experience of wonder filled me every time I entered the hedgerow as a child. I had no awareness of seeking God there, but the holy just found me. It had been way too long since I'd been there.

The pastor went on to say that there was something in every person so wonderful that only God could have put it there. That made me think about lots of people—my parents, Mother Phillips, and more. Intangible aspects of their lives and personalities couldn't be fully explained by psychology, sociology, nor any fancy college theories. Maybe, just maybe, God had something to do with it.

That night I knew something had changed way down deep inside me. I didn't know how to talk about it. Although Carole was still a teenager, she knew I needed to process whatever it was, so we went to see Mother Phillips—a remarkable lady from our church who was loved by the whole town. Her husband and children had died tragically, years before I'd met her. Instead of withdrawing from life and letting her pain make her bitter, she channeled the love she'd once lavished on her family and poured it into all the children of our town. She was one of the most faith-filled, delightful people I'd ever met.

Mother Phillips was very hard of hearing and her eyesight was dim but her spirit was totally alive and she could tell something major had happened to me. She was in her rocking chair when we let ourselves in. She took one look at me and opened her arms. She was a tiny, frail old woman. I was a college girl who snacked too much while I studied. But she rocked me as if I were a child. In that moment, I was a child. I opened my heart that night and somehow the God I thought I didn't need or even believe in anymore, became my heavenly Father. It paved the way for my later discoveries of Jesus as my Savior and of the power of the Holy Spirit.

AMBER'S STUFF

In February 1992, just about smack dab in the middle of the twilight years, my journal recorded wonder of a different kind—yet another memorable Communion service.

In his sermon, Dick explained in detail how he felt after Amber left. Our youngest, she was married right out of high school, and since her husband, Terry, was in the Navy, their early years were spent far from home, in Florida, West Virginia, and Italy. Dick talked about how he found her stuff in every room after she left, and of how she wrote long, descriptive letters. She called as often as she could too, with the result that her presence was still very much with us.

Then he said, "Just as Amber relates to us in many ways, so does Jesus. And Jesus is no more gone than Amber. You can't go anywhere without tripping all over his 'stuff.'"

I guess, for me, that's the most wonder-filled thing of all. Jesus is alive and it's his love, power, peace, and strength that made the waves of the twilight years shimmer with blessings. I didn't always see them at the time. Maybe you don't see them today. Keep looking for them, though. Keep trusting. Keep expecting. It could be that the rebirth of wonder in your life is just around the corner.

DICK'S GIFT TO ME

Dad died in that nursing home, and as it had been with Mom, I wasn't there. At first, it seemed so unfair that after all the years of caregiving I wasn't even given a decent goodbye. But then I realized we'd been saying goodbye to each other in lots of ways for a long, long time. Dad wasn't alone when the end came. Carole and John were there. More important, Jesus was there, the same Lord Dad had recognized in the back yard that day, four years before.

When Mom died, my cousin Kevin did the eulogy and Mom and Dad's pastor, Rod, did the funeral liturgy. Both men ministered to me. But when Dick offered to do Dad's service, I wanted and needed him to. I knew it wouldn't be easy for him, for many reasons.

He loved Dad very much, and was grieving with me. On October 22, 1994, Dick stood behind the pulpit in my home church in East Bloomfield, New York, and told stories about my precious father, Wes Ford, that made us laugh and cry.

Dick's closing words were the greatest gift of that hour. Tears are running down my cheeks now, as I share them with you:

> *Would you like to know the very best part? I have a vision I would like to share with you.*

I see Wes sitting in his wheelchair just outside the massive gate that leads into the Kingdom. In due course, he notices that he isn't slouched over to one side. Instead, his back is straight and his head is high. After a while, he tries the fingers of his left hand and they work. He tightens the muscles in his left shoulder, and his arm rises. He tries the toes and ankle of his left foot, and they move. He flexes the big muscles in his left thigh, and his knee bends.

And then, the limitless grace and the majestic power of God is evidenced again. Wes puts the palms of his hands on the arms of the chair, rises, and WALKS through the gate.

And all God's people said—Amen.

†·†·†

"Till I Reach the Promised Land"

Jesus makes even the most difficult caregiving days shimmer with blessings—but you must expectantly look for and claim those blessings!

Blessed be Jehovah God, the God of Israel, who only does wonderful things!

Psalm 72: 18

Prayer: *Father, I need you to restore the wonder I had as a child. Forgive me for ignoring the beauty you lavish all around me—especially in the people you've given me to care for.*

Shirl's Sanity Saver

Put on some beautiful music and let the melodies carry you into the presence of God. Stay there a while. Remember Corrie Ten Boom's words, "Don't wrestle; just nestle."

NOTES

Introductory Note: Dear Reader

1. Buck Ram: lyrics; Marty Nevens, Al Nevens, Artie Dunn: music,"Twilight Time," 1944. Nashville: EMI Music Publishing.

Chapter 2

1. TIAs: "Transient ischemic attacks (TIAs) are short-lived (lasting less than 24 hours) neurological deficits due to ischemia. An ischemic stroke occurs when blood flow is interrupted by blockage of an artery supplying blood to the brain. Most episodes subside within five to twenty minutes, they rarely continue for more than a few hours, and they are almost never painful. Hence, they tend to be ignored. TIAs are, however, an important warning sign of an impending stroke and thus warrant prompt medical attention.

   Possible warning signs:
   - sudden numbness, weakness or paralysis in the face or limbs (often on one side)
   - sudden loss, blurring, or dimness of vision
   - mental confusion, loss of memory or consciousness, unexplained drowsiness
   - slurred speech, loss of speech, difficulty in understanding others
   - sudden severe headache
   - unexplained dizziness, lack of coordination or fall
   - nausea and/or vomiting- especially with any of the symptoms above

If you or a loved one experiences these, seek medical help. Don't try to drive yourself to the ER. This information is from Simeon *The Johns Hopkins*

Medical Guide to Health After 50, by Simeon Marglois, M.D., PH.D., Medical ed. (New York: Medletter Associates, Inc., 2002)

But here is another bit of important information from Dr. Paul Donahue:

In his syndicated newspaper column, "To Your Health," Dr. Donahue gives this very important warning: "Most strokes are ischemic strokes- strokes due to obstruction of blood because of a clot in a brain artery. (Note from Shirl: That was my Dad's situation, and aspirin in the early days may have made a difference.) Twenty percent, however, are due to bleeding in the brain.

It's difficult to differentiate which kind of stroke a person has without a brain scan. Giving aspirin to a person who has had a brain bleed would almost seal the person's death. Clot-busting drugs are given in the ER. They don't prevent the clot from growing bigger, as aspirin does. They actually dissolve the clot." (April 10, 2011)

Chapter 3:

1. Elizabeth Payson Prentiss words. 1856 Howard Doane, music 1870, "More Love to Thee O Christ."

2. Dick and Melodie Tunney, "In His Presence," Lorenz Creative Services, 1988.

Chapter 11

1. Robert Robinson, "Come Thou Fount of Every Blessing," 1758.

Chapter 12

1. *Our Daily Bread*, Devotional publication from RBC ministries, Grand Rapids, MI, www.reb.org

2. Johnny Mercer (lyrics) and Henry Mancini (music) "Moon River," written by for the movie, *Breakfast at Tiffany's*, 1961.

Chapter 13

1. Norman Cousins, Anatomy of an Illness, (New York: W.W.W. Norton Co., 2005). Dr. Norman Cousins described how watching Marx Brothers movies helped him recover from a serious illness. He discovered that for him, a few minutes of laughter resulted in an hour or more of pain-free sleep.

Chapter 16

1. This was before the merger in 1968 with the E.U.B. that created the United Methodist Church.

2. Corrie ten Boom, *Don't Wrestle, Just Nestle*, (Old Tappan, N.J., Fleming H. Revell, 1978)

Chapter 17

1. Fynn, *Mr. God, This is Anna*, (London: William Collins Sons and Co Ltd., 1974).

Chapter 21

1. Home health aides: These angels of mercy come in many varieties, from experienced, professional RNs to those with little formal training, but a God-given compassion and a heart for caring. We used several sources to find our team, including the Office of the Aging, lists from local hospitals, and ads we placed in the paper. We interviewed more people than I can remember and discovered that formal training and education were not always the best criteria to hire someone. We knew what we

could afford per hour and worked from there, looking for strength of back, character, and heart more than advanced nursing degrees. Check references carefully and take advantage of the wonderful online resources available today.

2. The Holloway House Restaurant, Finger Lakes Dining, 29 State St, Rts. 5 and 20, East Bloomfield, New York. http//www.thehollowayhouse.com

3. Sally Lunn bread, "It is a rich round and generous brioche... similar to the historic French festival "breads." Sally Lunn was a Huguenot refugee. http.//www.sallylunns.com

Chapter 22

1. "Be Thou My Vision." Words: Attributed to Dallan Forgaill, 8th Century; translated from ancient Irish to English by Mary E. Byrne in *Eriú, Journal of the School of Irish Learning*, 1905, and versed by Eleanor H. Hull, 1912, alt. http://www.hymntime.com/tch/htm/b/e/t/bethoumv.htm

Chapter 23

1. Catherine Marshall, forward to *Beyond Ourselves,*(New York, McGraw-Hill Book Company, 1961) - and again in the forward to *Something More*, (New York- McGraw Hill Book Company- 1974).

Author Bio

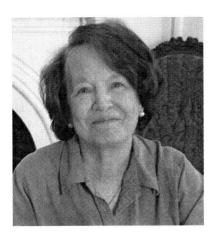

Shirley Leonard is a graduate of the Christian Writers Guild. Her devotionals have appeared in the *Secret Place, the Quiet Hour, Devotions,* and *Penned from the Heart.* Her short story, "Unexpected Shift," appeared in Live, and she's published articles in *Women Alive, Pennsylvania,* and *American Window Cleaner* magazines.

Shirley's caregiving experience spans four decades as a pastor's wife, including twenty years of nursing home ministry. She never imagined that one day her role would move from supporting church members who were caregivers to being a caregiver herself. After five years of taking care of her parents, she gained a new perspective on the needs of those she'd ministered to earlier. *With Each Passing Moment* is her story—a devotional memoir that reaches out to other caregivers—a story of finding help and hope in the Lord at a time when her human abilities and resources were exhausted.

For more information visit Shirley's web page at shirleysscene.com

CPSIA information can be obtained at www.ICGtesting.com
Printed in the USA
BVOW021655050313

314618BV00003B/5/P